Optimal
Men's Health

DR. WEIL'S HEALTHY LIVING GUIDES

Andrew Weil, MD, Series Editor

Integrative Medicine is healing-oriented medicine that takes account of the whole person, including all aspects of lifestyle. It emphasizes the therapeutic relationship between practitioner and patient, is informed by evidence, and makes use of all appropriate therapies.

Published and forthcoming titles:

Optimal Men's Health by Myles Spar
Non-Toxic: Living Healthy in a Chemical World by Aly Cohen
    and Frederick vom Saal
Optimal Aging by Mikhail Kogan
Optimal Skin Health by Robert Norman
Optimal Brain Health by Daniel Monti and Andrew Newberg

Optimal Men's Health

By
Myles Spar, MD, MPH
Founder and President, DrSpar.com
Chief Medical Officer,
Vault Health, Inc.

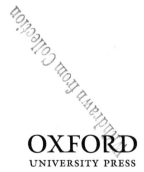

OXFORD
UNIVERSITY PRESS

OXFORD
UNIVERSITY PRESS

Oxford University Press is a department of the University of Oxford. It furthers
the University's objective of excellence in research, scholarship, and education
by publishing worldwide. Oxford is a registered trade mark of Oxford University
Press in the UK and certain other countries.

Published in the United States of America by Oxford University Press
198 Madison Avenue, New York, NY 10016, United States of America.

Library of Congress Cataloging-in-Publication Data
Names: Spar, Myles D., author.
Title: Optimal men's health / by Myles Spar, MD, MPH,
Founder and President, Tack180, Director of Integrative Medicine,
Southern California Men's Medical Group.
Description: New York : Oxford University Press, 2020. |
Series: Dr. Weil's healthy living guides |
Includes bibliographical references and index.
Identifiers: LCCN 2019027218 (print) | LCCN 2019027219 (ebook) |
ISBN 9780190654870 (paperback) | ISBN 9780190654894 (epub) |
ISBN 9780190654887 (updf)
Subjects: LCSH: Men—Health and hygiene.
Classification: LCC RA777.8 .S657 2020 (print) | LCC RA777.8 (ebook) |
DDC 613/.04234—dc23
LC record available at https://lccn.loc.gov/2019027218
LC ebook record available at https://lccn.loc.gov/2019027219

9 8 7 6 5 4 3 2 1

Printed by LSC Communications, United States of America

This book is dedicated to my teachers. By that, I mean my family, colleagues, professors, friends and patients—because my growth and learning has come through all of them. I offer this book as a tool to help men to become more engaged in their own health; thus I also dedicate it to anyone who gets something useful from these pages.

Contents

Section One: The Foundations of Optimal Health for Men

Section Two: Specific Male Health Goals: Prevention and Integrative Approach to Treatment

Section Three: Complementary Medicine and Men's Health

Section Four: Conclusion

Series Foreword

In 2013, I asked Dr. Myles Spar to be the senior co-editor of *Integrative Men's Health*, a volume in the Weil Integrative Medicine Library published by Oxford University Press. This was an academic work intended for health professionals. In the foreword I wrote for it, I stated my belief that it would give practitioners useful information and resources to provide better care for male patients. I could not have been more pleased with the book Dr. Spar produced.

Both he and I saw a need to make the information in it accessible to a general readership. Although men have unique health needs and their disease risks are different from those of women, most books and magazines addressing men's health focus narrowly on fitness. With the publication of *Optimal Men's Health*, there is now a resource that explains how the lifestyle choices men make influence both physical and emotional health and what men can do to achieve optimal well-being.

In these pages Dr. Spar gives you the facts and tools you need and, I hope, the motivation to put them to use.

Andrew Weil, MD
Tucson, Arizona
October 2019

Preface

It's hard to be a man.

I know that men aren't engendering a lot of sympathy these days, but the fact of the matter is that some of the reasons some men behave badly are also the reasons men are less healthy than women. The need to feel strong and the fear of being perceived as weak have undermined men's own self-interest. We all need to reach out to others—to share what concerns or scares us, to ask for help, to get support—but reaching out makes men feel weak, so they reach for a beer instead of a phone and go to a game instead of a doctor.

This book is not about teaching men to be vulnerable or getting men to share more. It is about men winning. Because winning requires teamwork and coaches and experts, and winning is not weak. Winning at what? That is up to you—but in my view, first and foremost, you need to be healthy in order to win, so this book is about starting there.

I wrote this book because there is nothing else out there for men who want to proactively take charge of their own health using the whole spectrum of tools that can prevent disease and maintain optimal health—an approach we call integrative medicine, because it integrates lifestyle, prevention approaches, pharmaceutical approaches, and non-Western approaches in a science-based and comprehensive way. Sure, there are books for men on fitness and on specific conditions. But this is your guide for winning at whatever matters most to you—not just building muscles or preventing one disease. It's about prevention and treatment of all of the most common diseases of concern to men, and it's about what tools you should have in your toolbox beyond simply pharmaceuticals.

You can read this book cover to cover or skip to a chapter that feels relevant. In order to win, you need practical tools—so each chapter ends with a quick "Bottom Line" section along with relevant resources and questions to ask your own healthcare practitioner, because I want to support that relationship with a doctor, not replace it.

In order to win, you need to change behavior as much as you need information. This book helps you with both. Reading it, you'll understand how much control you actually have over your own health, and what the next best steps are for you to take. Look at it as your guide to what to do to stay healthy and win.

Myles Spar, MD

Acknowledgments

Books are a labor of passion and take a village. I wrote this book because my "why" is to engage and equip men to be more proactive in their health, thereby making it more likely they will achieve their goals in general. Toward that end, I have garnered the help of many people along the way.

I especially want to thank Drs. Andrew Weil and Victoria Maizes from the University of Arizona Andrew Weil Center for Integrative Medicine. They have supported this "why" by allowing me to insert training for practitioners about how to truly reach men through the fellowship and this book. I also want to thank my colleagues in Integrative Medicine who have nurtured this passion about broadening our approach. I started my journey into integrative men's health alongside my colleague, Dr. Edison de Mello at the Akasha Center for Integrative Medicine in Santa Monica, so I owe him a debt of gratitude for being a pioneer in this field with me.

Thank you to my other colleagues in men's health including Joel Heidelbaugh and David Greenberg who have been true role models and colleagues in integrative medicine, Geeta Maker-Clark and Sara Gottfried, who generously showed how much they cared about me and my work. My Tack180 family also travelled this journey with me, and they cheered me on every step of the way, so to Jamie Eysenbach, Kiara Low Dog, and Allen Garcia I give much thanks.

The team at Oxford University Press has been so helpful and patient along the way, and I want to especially acknowledge and thank Andrea Knobloch, Amy Whitmer, and Emily Samulski for their encouragement and assistance.

Men often owe their good health to the women and role models in their life, and this is no less true for me. My sister, Mindy, has always been an unwavering source of love and support. My mother's care for my father has kept him going for many years through health challenges, and my dad's positive attitude about life has certainly influenced my own understanding of what it means to be a healthy man.

I'd especially like to thank my family, Danny, Clio, and Canaan, who have supported all of my professional endeavors with trust and unconditional love, even when it causes significant disruption to their lives. There aren't words for how much that means to me.

Myles Spar, MD
2019

Optimal
Men's Health

SECTION 1

The Foundations of Optimal Health for Men

1

The Unique Health Needs of Men

Men's health is more than the sum of all healthcare that is not specific to women. It is about addressing the health needs and concerns specific to men. In fact, maleness itself is a risk factor for premature death. It's a fact that men die younger than women, have higher rates of many serious, life-threatening diseases, and approach healthcare very differently than women do—as in they typically ignore it. In fact, men are half as likely to have a regular source of healthcare as women.

We take it for granted that women live longer than men. This is the case in over 98 percent of countries in the world. In the United States, average life expectancy is almost five years longer for women than for men (76.3 years for men vs. 81.1 years for women).[1] Almost five years! Why? Why is it that for every major cause of mortality that affects both men and women, men die faster?

Are men genetically programmed to die sooner than women? Is it determined in our genes that men develop cancer and heart disease more often than women? No. Men have a 60 percent higher chance of developing cancer and a 40 percent higher chance of dying from cancer than women, even when you leave out gender-specific cancers like breast, cervical, and prostate cancers. In fact, men have an increased risk of mortality, both cancer-related and non-cancer-related, at all ages. Of the top ten causes of death in the United States, men are winning in nine of them.

This difference in lifespan between men and women has been relatively unexamined because it has been assumed to be based on biology. But this does not appear to be the case. For one, the extent of the gender gap in life expectancy changes across time and across countries. In the United States, the gap has been narrowing, from 7.8 years in 1979 to 4.8 years in 2011. If the gender gap were encoded in our genes, it would not be changing so much over time. The change is thought to be due to women increasingly taking on stresses and habits that used to affect mostly men, such as smoking, drinking alcohol, and working outside the home, while men are still less likely to lead a health-promoting lifestyle. Clearly there is more to the gender gap than our genes.

Perhaps masculinity itself is killing us. It seems that doctor avoidance, risk-taking behavior, and stress may be the best explanations for the gender gap. It is true that men just don't go to the doctor. Men are twice as likely as women to say they do not have a usual source of healthcare, and men attend half as many preventive care visits. This means there are only half as many opportunities to screen men for high blood pressure, obesity, high cholesterol, high blood sugar, substance abuse, cigarette smoking, depression, and anxiety. Not identifying such risks means fewer chances to intervene in a disease process before it results in a heart attack, a stroke, diabetes, or cancer.

Male gender roles may play a part in making men feel that they should deal with symptoms or illness on their own. Just as men typically don't ask for directions when lost, they may feel it is not "masculine" to seek help for potentially serious medical symptoms. But it is not all us guys' fault—too often, the visit to our healthcare practitioner is perfunctory and unrevealing. The typical annual physical is unlikely to be beneficial, as has been shown by the U.S. Preventive Services Task Force. Some healthcare providers, such as myself, are offering more impactful prevention-oriented annual exams, but most are just not changing the way they do yearly checkups. Still, to the extent that higher mortality can be explained by avoidance of the healthcare system, it is important to make resources available that are more relevant, impactful, and accessible to men.

There is a need for an approach to men's health that addresses men's specific concerns, such as sexual function, prostate issues, avoidance of heart disease, and maintaining healthy weight and optimal performance, in a way that is responsive, approachable, and thorough. A precision prevention model that focuses on working with men to help them achieve their goals by facilitating optimal health does just that.

What does a precision prevention approach look like? It is essentially an integrative medicine model, which uses science-based methods, focuses on prevention and the influence of lifestyle on health, and is open to new and cutting-edge paradigms, combining conventional therapies with complementary and alternative therapies while seeking natural and safer health solutions individualized to the goals of each patient. This book takes such an approach, which involves the use of the most advanced assessments of a patient's current state of health and risks for future health problems, including genetic and other predictive testing.[2]

Just as important, it starts with a patient's goals rather than merely his chief complaints. After all, health is the most significant influence on whether or not a man is optimally positioned to achieve his goals, such as performance at work, in bed, or in the boardroom. In other words, most men respond better to recommendations around health behaviors that will help specifically with whatever goals matter to them, rather than an abstract goal of wellness. Specific goals that optimal health can foster might include being more energetic, being more "on" at work, being more sexually confident, looking better, or being a better father—so why not focus on such goals rather than a general concept of health solely for health's sake? It's much more motivating. When those goals are coupled with personalized risk assessments, the recommendations you get are much more likely to have an impact.

What Do You Want Your Health For?

When I am seeing a patient, I don't start by asking what health problems he has or recommend general tips for overall wellness. I start with "What do you want your health for?" and then craft a plan, given his current state, lab studies, genetic test results, risks, lifestyle, and goals, to make sure his health is optimally positioned to help him achieve those goals. Because the fact is that *when you're healthy, you can win.*

This approach empowers patients to actively participate in their health and healing by developing an understanding of all factors that influence health. It also motivates people to make the behavior changes being recommended—because it is about helping to reach goals, to win at what matters most, rather than simply not being sick.

This comprehensive approach utilizes various tools, or levers, to affect the overall health of a person. These tools of optimal health incorporate an integrative approach. All the levers can be used to varying degrees.

- *Medical.* This is the lever you're most familiar with from traditional doctor recommendations and tests, including the use of prescription and over-the-counter medications.
- *Nutrition.* Diet has a huge impact on health and is a powerful tool in your arsenal for achieving your goals.
- *Behaviors.* Drinking, smoking, and things that interfere with sleep, such as excessive screen time, can waylay the achievement of what's really important to you.
- *Stress and emotions.* Feeling depressed, anxious, or stressed likewise can prevent you from achieving even the most basic progress toward health and overall goals. But there are powerful tools available for minimizing their impact.
- *Social.* Engaging with a community, even one that fosters some competition, can be a very motivating and uplifting part of optimal health.
- *Physical activity.* Staying active is perhaps the most powerful anti-aging tool we have.
- *Spiritual.* This relates to having an identified goal or purpose. Feeling connected with some reason to pursue your goals is extremely motivating
- *Environment.* What and whom you surround yourself with can facilitate health—or add to your toxic burden.

How Can You Use These Tools to Your Advantage? Mike's Story

Mike was a typical patient of mine. When I spoke to Mike about losing weight in order to lessen the risk of problems like diabetes and heart disease and to optimize his overall wellness, I could see his eyes glaze over. I knew that the way I approached integrative medicine with women would not work with many guys. To generalize, men wait until something is broken before seeking help. The idea of putting out effort or sacrificing what they want to eat on the off chance it could improve something as intangible as wellness is less alluring to many men than it is to many women. Mike wasn't interested in optimizing some abstract concept or perhaps decreasing chances of some disease far in the future.

But Mike did want to coach his six-year-old son's soccer team, and he didn't have the stamina he needed to be able to do a decent job at it. He wanted to know what he needed to do to get there. Aha! I had something to work toward—better health for a purpose that was personal and relevant to Mike.

Mike taught me that I needed to change the way I approach many of my male patients. Now I ask, "What are your goals?" Not exactly what patients are used to hearing in the annual physical from their doctor! But these goals frame the whole visit—the initial examination, the tests I choose to do, and the recommendations I ultimately make.

In fact, having a goal or a sense of purpose actually increases lifespan. In a systematic review of ten prospective studies enrolling a total of over 130,000 people, having a sense of purpose significantly reduced mortality and risk of cardiovascular events like heart attacks.[3] Yes, you read that right—identifying a clear reason for getting up in the morning decreased the chance of death by 17 percent.

When I ask patients what their goals are, many haven't really thought about it before. Mike was easy—he was clear that he wanted to coach his son's team. That drive increases his health and even his longevity. And studies show that clarity of purpose makes it more likely he will achieve his goals. Plus it gives me something concrete to work with.

For Mike, I was able to craft a plan around the eight levers that would maximize his chance of getting into better shape. These eight levers are what will be used throughout this book to frame approaches to specific medical conditions and health approaches that are most relevant to men's health. Let's look at how each lever provides approaches that can contribute to helping optimize Mike's health in order for him to achieve his goals. The following chapters in Section One will elaborate on each of these levers, but for Mike specifically, here is what they meant.

Medical. This encompasses much of what we think of as general Western medicine—determining what impacts health in men and figuring out what to look for in assessing a patient. It turned out that Mike had low thyroid hormone levels, so I started him on a low dose of thyroid hormone to help his energy, which should also help him to lose weight.

Nutritional. This encompasses not only diet but also nutritional supplements. Mike needed to lose weight to help his stamina and fitness, so I recommended a diet that matched his genetic type and supplements like L-carnitine, ginseng, and coenzyme Q10 to help with energy.

Exercise. To increase stamina, Mike needed a training program that gradually increased in intensity or incorporated interval training to improve his endurance and help him lose weight.

Behavioral. Mike had some habits that were interfering with his ability to get the most from the exercise program. For example, he played video games late at night, which stimulated his brain, making it harder to fall asleep and reducing his sleep to six hours a night. Lack of sleep not only decreased his energy but made it harder to lose weight and made him crave carbohydrates for energy, which resulted in sugar crashes that decreased his stamina. We discussed changing when and where he plays video games, agreeing that he'd stop one hour before a predetermined bedtime. This also helped his relationship with his wife—an added bonus.

Psychological. Mike had motivation. He didn't have significant psychological blocks to manifesting his vision, but he did get easily stressed out. When he was stressed from work, he would eat whatever was around and get off track from his exercise plan. So we worked on a stress management plan that incorporated mindfulness-based stress reduction—a sort of nonreligious meditation that helped Mike train himself to be more responsive to stressful situations and less reactive. This helped him to be less quick to grab a snack when stressed out.

Social and spiritual. Mike's primary motivation was social, and his family provided him with a strong sense of connection and purpose. Studies show that these will help him to achieve his goals. We will explore more on the impact of social connections and spiritual beliefs on health in the coming chapters.

Environmental. Mike brought his lunch to work every day in plastic containers to heat up in the microwave. The heated plastic releases pthalates into the food. Pthalates have been shown to lower testosterone.[4] Lower testosterone is associated with fatigue and weight gain, among other symptons, making it harder to lose weight. I suggested he switch to glass or ceramic containers, to help minimize hormonal effects that would interfere with achieving his goals.

The remaining chapters in this section will drill down further into each of these levers, using patient examples to show their major influence on health and how an integrative approach—one that starts with the identification of measurable goals and is accompanied by the use of an advanced personalized health assessment—creates real change.

Section Two will focus on specific health conditions of most concern to men, explaining how you can use this approach yourself to reach your health goals even when these conditions are present. This section is especially important for men looking to age more optimally; to perform better at work, in sports, and sexually; and to keep their brains sharp and focused.

Section Three takes you through complementary modalities that have solid scientific bases to their usefulness, explaining how they can impact the conditions most relevant to men and how to use them in conjunction with standard Western medicine.

Each chapter of this book provides resources you can use to incorporate this integrative medicine approach into your life to optimize your health and reach your goals. Health can be your greatest hurdle or your greatest source of strength. This book helps to make sure it is the latter.

For chapters where it's relevant, I've also included questions you may want to consider asking your primary care provider. For ease, I use the phrase "ask your doctor," but I realize your primary care provider may be a nurse practitioner or other healthcare provider.

The Bottom Line

Achieving optimal health is the most important factor in reaching your goals, and you have many ways to do this besides medications. The approach in this book is an integrative one, based on precision prevention: what can get in the way of staying healthy, and what you can do about it, from diet and exercise to supplements and meditation.

Notes

1. Kenneth D. Kochanek, Sherry L. Murphy, and Jiaquan Xu, "Deaths: Final Data for 2011," *National Vital Statistics Report* 63, no. 3 (July 27, 2015), http://www.cdc.gov/nchs/data/nvsr/nvsr63/nvsr63_03.pdf.
2. "Precision medicine" is a newer term frequently associated with treatment of serious illness, such as cancer, utilizing a personalized approach that targets therapies at an individual's unique cancer type. However, precision medicine can also be used as a prevention technique, incorporating an assessment of unique health risks based on personal health history, current lifestyle, and genetic testing and involving the development of a personalized plan for disease prevention and optimal health maintenance.
3. R. Cohen, C. Bavishi, and A. Rozanski, "Purpose in Life and Its Relationship to All-Cause Mortality and Cardiovascular Events: A Meta-Analysis," *Psychosomatic Medicine* 78, no. 2 (February–March 2016): 122–133, doi: 10.1097/PSY.0000000000000274.

4. John D. Meeker and Kelly K. Ferguson, "Urinary Phthalate Metabolites Are Associated with Decreased Serum Testosterone in Men, Women, and Children from NHANES 2011–2012," *Journal of Clinical Endocrinology and Metabolism* 99, no. 11 (2014): 4346–4352, doi: 10.1210/jc.2014-2555.

2

Optimal Health Assessment for Men

The first lever that we have in both assessing and influencing health is the one we call *medical*. This is the way of diagnosing and treating illness that we are most used to experiencing in the American health care system. But this approach all too often relies on waiting until disease presents itself with symptoms and then putting out fires with prescription medications, as opposed to preventing them in the first place or at least smelling for smoke before real damage occurs. The integrative approach to optimal health relies on using medications as needed and as an important treatment, but as a sort of last resort—when attempts at prevention or early intervention have failed.

Optimal Health Starts with an Optimal Medical Assessment

So, how do we decide what an individual person can do to prevent disease—or even how to prevent problems that interfere with his ability to pursue his goals? Of course, there are general recommendations that nearly everyone should follow in order to stay healthy, such as engaging in regular physical activity and eating a healthy diet. But what does that mean specifically for you? And what more can you do to stay healthy?

The most powerful strategies to prevent problems are the most specific, targeting your risks for disease depending on what particular health conditions you already have, your family history and genetics, and your lifestyle (including general dietary habits, exercise regimen, and any sleep or stress issues). Your annual physical, or checkup, is the perfect time to get tests that can identify some of your risks. But studies actually show that the typical annual checkup is ineffective at preventing disease or even death.[1] That's because the same generic tests are done on everyone, regardless of individual risk factors. The routine tests in an annual physical are geared toward finding out if anything is already wrong—with your kidneys or liver, for example—as opposed to trying to predict what could go wrong in the future. This is the opposite of personalized, prevention-oriented medicine. Certainly it's important to find out if your cholesterol or blood sugar is high. But there are other tests, ones often not done in a typical insurance-based annual physical, that can be even more significant for your individual health situation. And the tests that are currently routinely done are not as predictive for risk of future disease as we would like to believe, while more advanced testing is available but not routinely used. Do you know that most major heart attacks occur in people with normal cholesterol? Clearly there are better predictive tests we can be using.

We have entered an age of more personalized medicine, called precision medicine, and this needs to be applied to prevention as well as the treatment of disease. The generic annual checkup that uses the same tests for everyone, regardless of particular risks or goals, is becoming an anachronism. This chapter will review some of the more detailed assessments that can be done to better equip you with actionable information to stay on your game.

Why do these more detailed measurements make a difference? Let's look at two examples of guys who have the same findings on the generic annual checkup but have very different risks for heart attacks based on more advanced predictive testing.

Pete and Dave: Same Cholesterol Levels, Different Risks

Pete and Dave are the same age. Both of them try to eat well. Both play basketball. Both have a family history of early heart disease (a grandfather with a heart attack in his early fifties). In fact, they get the same reports from their doctors—that their cholesterol is a little high and they need to lose a few pounds, but otherwise there are no red flags. The results of their standard lab tests are nearly identical. So why does Pete actually have a much higher risk of having a heart attack?

If these guys had a more precision, prevention-oriented annual physical, it might include genetic testing for ApoE, a gene that can confer higher risk of heart disease and Alzheimer's if present in a specific variation (ApoE4). It turns out that Pete does have two copies of ApoE4, increasing by a factor of over ten his risk for heart disease at a young age. An expanded prevention-oriented exam might also include a coronary calcium CT scan; Pete's showed plaque in the arteries around his heart, while Dave's did not. And this advanced testing would include C-reactive protein, a marker of inflammation proven to correlate with higher risk of heart disease, and which is higher in Pete than in Dave.

Both of these gentlemen would be treated the same way if only the typical annual physical is done—for example, both would be counseled to eat a diet lower in saturated fat. But because the true increased risk for Pete wouldn't be recognized, that recommendation wouldn't suffice, and Pete might well have a heart attack before he turns fifty.

Table 2.1 Generic Annual Physical Versus an Optimal Health Assessment

	Traditional Checkup	Precision Prevention-Oriented Optimal Health Assessment
Orientation	Focused on your chief complaints	Focused on your goals
Sample tests*	Metabolic panel, lipids, blood count, TSH	Metabolic panel, lipids, blood count, TSH, free hormone levels, vitamin levels, Advanced lipid panel, calcium score, ApoE, MTHFR
Recommendations	Medications	Medications
	General diet	Supplements
		Specific nutritional recommendations
		Use of complementary modalities
		Stress management
		Sleep hygiene recommendations

* More details on testing are shown in Table 2.2.

Precision Tests

CRP

With the goal of optimal health and prevention, we can use advanced testing to drill deeper and identify risks one man may have that another doesn't. Table 2.1 shows the more in-depth detail that an optimal prevention-oriented personalized health checkup can provide. For example, a prevention-oriented set of labs should include a check for inflammation markers, like C-reactive protein (CRP). Why is this? We used to think that the circulatory system was like plumbing, and that a heart attack happened when the arteries that supply blood, and therefore oxygen, to the heart muscle get clogged up with plaque, blocking the flow of blood completely. In fact, this is not the case—it became clear that some people had high rates of blockage (called stenosis) without having heart attacks, while others had relatively little blockage but would go on to have a heart attack. What we discovered was that arterial blockage is about more than plaque buildup—it's about plaque that is inflamed and therefore prone to rupture, causing a blood clot to form at the site of the plaque. *That's* when the blood stops flowing to the heart, causing a heart attack. So "the big one" requires this lethal combination of cholesterol plaque plus inflammation.

SNPs

New, widely available genetic testing can detect genetic variations, called SNPs, that are in our DNA.[2] SNPs, or single nucleotide polymorphisms, are a variation in the sequence (the pattern) of DNA that occurs in some people, resulting in a difference in what the DNA tells the cell to do.[3] For example, DNA that codes for proteins involved in cholesterol metabolism may have a variation in the sequence of its nucleotides such that people with that variation are more likely to have different issues with cholesterol than people without that SNP.

Some SNPs are associated with risks of various diseases. Take the ApoE gene, mentioned earlier in this chapter. Remember, genes are just a bunch of DNA that codes for a particular characteristic. The ApoE gene provides instructions for making a protein called apolipoprotein E. This protein combines with fats (lipids) in the body to form molecules called lipoproteins. Lipoproteins are responsible for packaging cholesterol and other fats and carrying them through the bloodstream. Variations in this gene affect the function of these lipoproteins, such that people with the

ApoE4 form of the gene make a form of apolipoprotein that is more likely to cause plaques. There are three variations of this gene that are found in humans: ApoE2, ApoE3, and ApoE4. Each one has a slightly different sequence of nucleotides, and each one causes apolipoprotein E to behave a little differently. The most prevalent form of this gene is ApoE3. With genes, we get one copy from our mother and one copy from our father. If you have one copy of ApoE2, you have a 40 percent lower risk of both heart disease and Alzheimer's; the decrease in risk is even greater if you have two copies. If you have the ApoE4 variant, however, your risk for both conditions is *increased*. If you have one copy of ApoE4 and one copy of the more prevalent ApoE3 gene, your risk is increased two- or threefold. If you have two copies of ApoE4, your risk is increased twelvefold.

MTHFR

Another important genetic test looks at the genes associated with MTHFR, or methylenetetrahydrofolate reductase, an enzyme that is needed for methylation—a chemical reaction necessary for proteins to function well and for DNA to work normally. Good methylation is key to a strong immune system and detoxification. If your MTHFR enzyme is not working well, you have a hard time clearing dangerous substances from your body. Abnormal function of MTHFR is associated with heart disease, inflammation, dementia, chronic fatigue, and buildup of toxins.

There are two genes with SNPs that affect this enzyme's activity.[4] Normally functioning MTHFR genes produce enough enzyme to facilitate the conversion of folate into a more usable form, L-methylfolate. Folate is an essential B vitamin that helps turn amino acids into compounds like serotonin and dopamine. The most widely known consequence of having mutations in one or both MTHFR genes is that you have a diminished ability to turn the dangerous amino acid homocysteine into the benign amino acid methionine. When homocysteine builds up, it significantly increases the risk of plaque buildup in the arteries around the heart. Forty percent of people have at least one defective MTHFR gene; it is important to know if you are in this group.

Epigenetics, or Why It Is Helpful to Know Your Genes

When I was in medical school in the 1990s, we were taught that people were basically victims of their genetic inheritance. Everyone gets one copy of each gene from their biological mother and one copy from their biological father. "Bad" genes, we learned, could increase risk for all sorts of health problems, from heart disease to diabetes and autoimmune illnesses like lupus and asthma. Under this scenario, the only reason to get one's genes tested would be to be able to intervene early. If I knew I was at risk for diabetes from my genes, for example, I might start minimizing sugar in my diet in order to delay or prevent a diabetes diagnosis.

But over the last twenty-five years, we have discovered that not everyone with the gene that puts them at risk for diabetes actually develops the condition. It has been shown that what we do and eat, our life experiences and exposures, and even what we think influence how genes are expressed— that is, which genes get turned on and which get turned off. You may inherit a gene that puts you at higher risk of prostate cancer, but you can lessen your chance of getting prostate cancer by turning off that gene. How we turn genes on and off is called epigenetics.

What controls gene expression? Actually, a lot of things. When it comes to oncogenes—genes that, when turned on, code for proteins that increase risk of cancer—we know that diet, stress, and physical activity all influence whether these genes get turned on or not. In fact, real, consistent lifestyle change not only turns genes on and off for you but also affects to some extent how genes will be turned on or off in your future children and grandchildren. The mechanism through which this happens is DNA methylation, the same process described in the section about the MTHFR gene—a biochemical process of adding a methyl group to the DNA molecule, which serves to switch genes on or off.[5] A study of people with stomach cancer showed that participants could affect methylation of an important gene involved in their cancer by drinking green tea and eating cruciferous vegetables. Research shows that methylation is even affected by environmental factors such as exposure to pollutants and overall stress.

This means that the power to control your genetic health is, to an extent, in your hands—if you're willing to be proactive about lifestyle changes like eating well, exercising, and managing stress. Just because your grandfather and father suffered a certain fate doesn't mean you will, too.

Back to Pete and Dave. Because we were able to use precision medical testing to determine that, despite having the same cholesterol levels, Pete has plaque in his arteries, higher inflammation, and more unfavorable genes, while Dave has no evidence of plaque, lower inflammation,

Table 2.2 Testing Done in the Generic Annual Physical and in an Optimal Health Assessment

Ask your primary care practitioner about whether some of these tests may be right for you.

Typical Annual Physical	Precision Prevention Physical
Metabolic panel, CBC	Metabolic panel, CBC
Standard lipid panel: total cholesterol, LDL, HDL, triglycerides	Advanced lipid panel: total cholesterol, LDL, HDL, triglycerides, particle sizes, CRP, homocysteine, Lp(a), ApoB
Blood sugar: glucose	Metabolic risk assessment: glucose, insulin, leptin, hemoglobin A1C
Thyroid screen: TSH	Thyroid in-depth assessment: TSH, free T3, free T4, reverse T3, thyroid antibodies
Vitamin D	Multiple vitamin levels
	Genetic testing
	Heart scan for calcium score
	Artery scan for plaque
	Bone scan for bone density and body composition
	Telomeres for cellular aging
	Oxidative stress test
	Adrenal/cortisol test
	Full hormone assessment
Cancer risk screening: PSA	PSA, cancer gene testing (depending on individual risk)

and more favorable genes, we would treat the two of them very differently. Pete should have more aggressive treatment to control his higher risk of heart disease. We will discuss in Chapter 7 what sort of treatment is appropriate for preventing heart attacks in someone at high risk, but in summary, Pete's optimal heart attack prevention plan would include a statin drug plus personalized dietary recommendations, supplement suggestions, and stress management tips.

Dave, who has high cholesterol but no evidence of plaque, can safely continue without a statin. For him we'd recommend some dietary changes, an omega-3 supplement, the right exercise program, and a stress management program. So despite the same general test results, Pete and Dave require very different preventative regimens in order to have the best chance of avoiding heart attack and stroke.

The point here is that we can find preclinical disease (meaning abnormalities that are detectable before they cause any symptoms or any abnormalities on the standard annual lab work) and intervene *before* actual disease starts. And there is very strong evidence that certain lifestyle behaviors, supplements, and diets can alter the course of health and possibly even allow you to avoid taking medications, which generally cost more and have more side effects than simple lifestyle changes or nutritional supplements.

So now we have a much broader and more powerful set of tools that we can use to check on your health, assess your risk of future health problems, and decide how to intervene in order to minimize the chance of such problems developing. For example, the optimal men's health assessment (see Table 2.2) is a precision tool that includes all the basics checked for in the standard annual physical and adds to it tests that help identify what may need to be done to prevent future problems. We look at advanced measures of risk for heart disease and metabolic disease, genetic factors influencing disease risk, and nutritional status by measuring micronutrient levels. We also test the strength of the immune system and the body's ability to withstand oxidative damage, among other things. The specific tests that will be recommended will depend each person's unique goals, past medical history, family history, and current diseases or symptoms.

Tim: Brain Health Issues

Tim, fifty-three, is worried because his mom has Alzheimer's. He is beginning to notice some memory issues in himself, and he wants to do everything he can to avoid getting the dementia he sees destroying his mother.

> *Tests that can help assess Tim's risk:* ApoE gene variants, CRP (inflammation marker), lipid peroxides (oxidative stress marker), blood sugar testing, vitamin level testing
>
> *Interventions that can help Tim decrease his risk:* adding supplements to decrease inflammation; optimizing his diet to minimize processed foods, added sugars, inflammation-promoting foods, and possibly gluten; engaging in regular physical activity; limiting alcohol; taking brain-protective supplements like acetyl-L-carnitine, omega-3 fatty acids, and nootropics

This is what the modern medical assessment for optimal health should do: empower people to be proactive in preventing problems that can interfere with the ability to do what matters to them—to be active and effective at work, at play, and with their family and friends.

The Bottom Line

I recommend this broad array of tests and a panoply of interventions because the optimal health tool kit is about more than medications. Now we have so many more ways than before to assess your risks of serious health problems and to mitigate those risks. These are science-based approaches that you can implement right away—they go beyond simply taking medications to include lifestyle changes such as diet, exercise, and stress management.

Action Plan: Preparing for Your Next Annual Physical

1. Take a few minutes to write down what you want your health *for*. When you go to your appointment, share this with your provider so she knows what matters *to* you, not just what's the matter *with* you.
2. Ask about any tests that are not part of the routine checkup but which could help you and your provider better understand what changes you should make in your diet, supplement regimen, exercise program, or other lifestyle habits in order to avoid having health problems interfere with your life.
3. Ask about genetic testing and other testing (see Table 2.2) to better home in on your particular risk of disease.
4. If a new medication is recommended, ask if there are things you could *safely* do with diet, exercise, supplements, or use of complementary modalities before adding that medication.

Notes

1. Ateev Mehrota and Allan Prochazka, "Improving Value in Health Care—Against the Annual Physical," *New England Journal of Medicine* 373 (2015): 1485–1487, doi: 10.1056/NEJMp1507485.
2. Genetic testing options are changing rapidly. There are direct-to-consumer tests available online starting at $99. More robust tests cost more, of course, and the best tests are available through practitioners who can help to interpret the results and provide recommendations based on those results. But insurance may or may not cover these tests, which for multiple genes can run from $300 to over $500.
3. Nucleotides are the building blocks of DNA. There are four of them: adenine (A), guanine (G), cytosine (C), and thymine (T). DNA carries the instructions for every cell in our body. If a piece of DNA is responsible for telling the body how to handle cholesterol, then a difference in the sequence of nucleotides that make up that piece of DNA will give the body different instructions for handling cholesterol than would be seen in people without that variation in the nucleotide sequence.

4. The two genes that impact MTHFR activity are called C677T (where thymine replaces the normal cytosine at the 677th position on the DNA strip) and A1289C (where cytosine replaces adenine at the 1289th position).
5. Methylation adds a methyl group—one carbon atom and three hydrogen atoms—to proteins. When the methyl group is added (or removed, in demethylation) from parts of DNA called histones, the amount of protein that chunk of DNA normally makes increases or decreases.

3

What to Eat
for Optimal Health

Arguably the most powerful lever that influences health and risk for disease is diet. We know that diet can play an important role in lessening risk for disease, as seen from the evidence of decreased risk for many cancers from eating more fruits, vegetables, and fiber, while eating poorly can increase disease risk significantly, such as when eating too much sugar and processed foods leads to metabolic syndrome or diabetes. But those are extreme and perhaps obvious examples. When it comes to overall health and disease prevention, why is there such contradictory information about which diets are best? When there are so many diets being touted for various health benefits—paleo, Mediterranean, ketogenic, vegan, low-fat—what should men eat?

The first and most important fact is that any healthy diet minimizes processed foods, typical snack foods, and added sugars, especially sugar-sweetened beverages. These foods have been definitively associated with weight gain and the development of diseases associated with obesity, like diabetes and heart disease. Specifically, potato chips, white potatoes in general, sugar-sweetened beverages (soda, energy drinks, sweet tea, sugary coffee drinks), and both processed and unprocessed red meats were associated with weight gain in a large study of over 120,000 healthy men and women spanning twenty years. Foods shown to be associated with weight loss were vegetables, whole grains, fruits, nuts, and yogurt.[1]

Processed foods are generally less healthy, but what exactly are processed foods? Basically, they are anything that is made in a manufacturing plant, involving artificial ingredients or the use of chemical processes to change or preserve the food. Some of the most infamous manufactured food components are the hydrogenated oils, known as trans fats. These have actually been banned by the FDA. Other processed foods may not be so obvious: think of corn chips instead of corn, or instant oatmeal with sugar and flavorings instead of whole oats. The less a food looks like it did in its natural form, the more processed it is. So making these basic changes away from processed foods, added sugars, and saturated fats is the first step away from the standard American diet, or SAD, and it will serve you well in avoiding the fate of the majority of Americans.

Anti-Inflammatory Diet

Beyond these basics, there is good evidence that, in terms of prevention of diseases such as obesity, diabetes, heart disease, cancer, and neurocognitive decline associated with aging, the overall best course is an anti-inflammatory diet.[2] This is largely because one commonality among these diseases is the process of inflammation itself. Anti-inflammatory diets emphasize plant-based foods like fruits, vegetables, whole grains, and beans, plus fish, while limiting the amount of meat and poultry consumed. This diet emphasizes healthy fats such as olive oil, nuts and seeds, and avocado; these contain high levels of healthful monounsaturated fat, which, along with omega-3 fatty acids, helps to alleviate inflammation. Inflammation is the process behind many medical conditions, from heart disease to autoimmune conditions to aging in general. This diet is very similar to what is known as a Mediterranean diet. Dr. Andrew Weil's anti-inflammatory pyramid illustrates the distribution of these foods on a daily and weekly basis (Figure 3.1).

If you want to keep it simple, you can stop reading now—for the average person, the anti-inflammatory diet is smart and preventive. But no one is average, and everyone has their own goals and risks. For example, if you've already had a heart attack, you would need to go deeper into a heart disease reversal approach and an aggressive anti-inflammatory lifestyle, getting stricter on your diet and possibly adding in supplements. In addition to eating a generally prevention-oriented diet, you would also focus

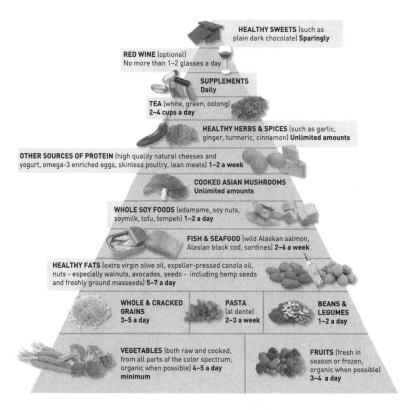

FIGURE 3.1 The Weil Anti-Inflammatory Pyramid

on other specific concerns, such as making sure the food you eat helps to control blood pressure and cholesterol.

Unfortunately, beyond the anti-inflammatory diet, there are many differing and even opposing recommendations. Take Pete and Dave, whom we met in Chapter 2. Dave may feel better and lose weight on a low-carb paleo-style diet, while Pete may have better success on a very low-fat diet. Why is that? Everyone is different, genetically and metabolically; hormones, metabolism, and the gastrointestinal system work somewhat differently in each of us. It's tough to know which diet is best for you—are you more like Dave or are you more like Pete? One way to tell is through genetic testing, as described in Chapter 2. Some tests can check which SNPs you have, and that can suggest which of your metabolic pathways could be functionally less than optimal. This would help your doctor to know which general diet or macronutrient profile is best for you.

Often, though, with or without genetic information, you know which sort of diet makes you feel better and helps you to accomplish your goals, whether it's to lose weight, feel more energetic, decrease gastrointestinal symptoms, or lower markers for disease risk such as cholesterol or blood sugar. The most important way to pick which diet is best for you is to examine your own unique health history, family history, lifestyle, and health concerns. In this chapter, we'll go through a brief rundown of various diets and the general conditions they have been shown to help, to try to help clarify some of the confusion. You can see some of these dietary differences in Table 3.1.

Paleo Diet

The paleo diet has become very popular. It is based on the idea that our diets should resemble the popular interpretation of how our caveman ancestors ate. The focus is on grass-fed beef, fish and other seafood, fruits and vegetables, eggs, nuts and seeds, and healthy oils, while minimizing refined vegetable oils and salt and avoiding all grains, legumes, refined sugars, potatoes, processed foods, and dairy. Some people do feel better on this diet and have luck losing weight, mostly because of the limited carbohydrate intake.

But there are problems with the underlying assumptions of this diet. First of all, newer studies have shown that our Paleolithic ancestors ate a mostly plant-based diet.[3] Second, there is evidence that they did eat processed grains and even types of flatbread. Third, while one of the main arguments made by enthusiasts of the paleo approach is that this diet must be beneficial because our Paleolithic ancestors did not suffer from the high levels of disease, like heart disease, that we currently do, actually evidence confirms that in fact they did have such disease when they died. Furthermore, there were multiple types of diets prevalent during the Paleolithic era, depending on location and food availability.

In fact, one problem with the paleo diet is its emphasis on meat and the exclusion of whole grains and legumes, which have health benefits. Research has consistently shown associations between high consumption of meat and incidence of heart disease, type 2 diabetes, high blood pressure, metabolic syndrome, and certain types of cancer.[4] People on the paleo diet may thrive merely because they are switching from the standard

Table 3.1 A Comparison of Popular Diets

Diet Type	Paleo	Low-Carb/Ketogenic	Low-Fat	Plant-Based	Intermittent Fasting
General	"Caveman" diet	Very low in carbs	Very low in fat	Whole plant-based foods	Avoid food for intermittent periods
Best for	Weight loss for some	Weight loss for some; beneficial for some neurological issues	Heart disease prevention and reversal	Cancer prevention, heart disease prevention and reversal	Longevity
Examples	Paleo, CrossFit	Keto, modified Atkins, South Beach	Dean Ornish	Vegan, vegetarian	5:2 diet, 8-Hour Diet, Fasting Mimicking Diet
People for whom it's not recommended		People with high cholesterol			People with blood sugar issues

Western processed diet to one that includes more whole foods. After all, there is much overlap with the anti-inflammatory diet, which promotes vegetables, fruits, nuts, and seeds, while minimizing processed foods and refined sugar.

One piece of advice I like about the paleo diet comes from the British National Health Service: "If you want to copy your Paleolithic ancestors, you're better off mimicking their activity levels rather than their alleged diet."[5] This means that, in an age where we are sitting in front of computers for most of the day, everyone will benefit from getting up and moving more. The promise of this diet just hasn't been borne out in terms of its historical accuracy or health benefits.

Low-Fat Diet

The low-fat diet has been championed and tested by Dr. Dean Ornish. In his Lifestyle Heart Trial, he showed that a comprehensive lifestyle change program including a low-fat diet led to about the same level of regression of arterial plaque (atherosclerosis) and decrease in bad cholesterol as that achieved by statin drugs, but it is hard to tell how much of the impact was from the diet and how much from the other facets of this program.[6] The Ornish Lifestyle Medicine program includes a very low-fat, mostly plant-based diet, regular exercise, group support, and a stress management program. In the diet, 10 percent of calories come from fat, 15–20 percent come from protein, and 70–75 percent come from carbohydrates, primarily fruits, vegetables, and whole grains.

This type of diet may be best for those who have preexisting heart disease or are at high risk for developing it, especially when it is used as part of a comprehensive lifestyle change. The overall program has even been shown to impact genetic expression (see Chapter 2) and the biological age of our cells, as measured by the length of telomeres (see https://www.ornish.com/wp-content/uploads/Lancet_Lifestyle-changes-lengthen-telomeres.pdf). Telomeres are structures at the ends of our DNA molecules that help to determine how many more times our cells can divide. As telomeres shrink, our cells can divide fewer times, so assessing the length of telomeres is a way to check how "old" the DNA in our cells is. For example, toxins shrink telomeres.

Actually, the low-fat diet Ornish recommends has much overlap with the Mediterranean diet in its emphasis on plant-based foods, minimally processed foods, and the inclusion of healthy grains, beans, and legumes, but it can be hard to follow with its very strict limit on all fat intake. The typical Mediterranean diet allows for a greater amount of healthy fats (especially monounsaturated and polyunsaturated fats).

Ketogenic or Low-Carb Diets

There are several versions of low-carb diets, including ketogenic diets and the Atkins diet. These are touted mostly for their impact on weight loss and some neurological issues. They all emphasize eliminating refined and simple carbohydrates and added sugars, which means that all packaged foods, juices, many fruits, white rice, bread, potatoes, and tortillas are off the menu. The idea is that reducing carbohydrate intake enough will force the body to shift from using carbohydrates (especially glucose) to using fat as a source of fuel, helping you to lose weight. Studies of these diets have not shown results as strong as those of the Mediterranean diet or low-fat diets for overall heart disease, diabetes, or cancer prevention, but some have shown an advantage to these diets for fat loss.

A ketogenic diet has been shown to be useful for certain neurological conditions, such as epilepsy and cognitive diseases ranging from mild cognitive impairment to Parkinson's disease and Alzheimer's. It is even being studied for autism and for degenerative diseases like ALS (amyotrophic lateral sclerosis, also known as Lou Gehrig's disease). There is mounting evidence that the classic ketogenic diet, as well as variations such as the modified Atkins diet, the MCT (medium-chain triglyceride) diet, and caloric restriction, has neuroprotective effects by repairing the function of mitochondria, the powerhouses that are in all our cells but are especially important in the brain. I'll go into more detail on the exciting new research into the impact of a ketogenic diet on recovery from neurological damage in Chapter 12.

Just cutting back on grains can help many people with both weight loss and brain health. Dr. David Perlmutter, a leading integrative neurologist, wrote extensively on the evidence linking grain consumption to poor brain health in his book *Grain Brain*. While whole grains are important parts of the anti-inflammatory and Ornish low-fat diets, Perlmutter emphasizes the impact of modern genetically modified grains on our gut and how that affects our brain, since we have a large network of neurons surrounding our alimentary canal. He argues that eating genetically modified grains treated with the weedkiller glyphosate causes a syndrome called "leaky gut" by damaging the normal populations of health-promoting bacteria that we have and need in our guts to help with digestion. Those healthy bacteria are essential to making sure we absorb the nutrients we need and keep out the things we don't want in our circulation. When that barrier gets disturbed, we end up absorbing things we shouldn't, which results in allergies, inflammation, and autoimmune conditions.

If weight loss or the prevention or treatment of neurological disease is your primary goal, it might be worth a try at the ketogenic diet, as long as carbs are replaced by healthier fats and proteins, not high amounts of saturated animal fat (an increase in heart disease is a concern on diets that promote sausages and bacon in lieu of toast, such as Atkins). The recommended ketogenic diets eliminate processed foods and promote high-quality fats from plants, wild-caught fish, organic poultry, and grass-fed beef, keeping saturated animal fat intake relatively low. For weight loss or increased energy, some people do benefit from cycling on and off a ketogenic diet within these parameters, but unless you have a neurological condition, it is rarely wise to stay on a ketogenic diet all the time. There simply aren't studies on the long-term effect of staying in a keto state indefinitely, as there are for plant-based and anti-inflammatory diets.

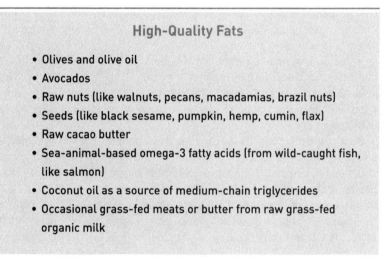

High-Quality Fats

- Olives and olive oil
- Avocados
- Raw nuts (like walnuts, pecans, macadamias, brazil nuts)
- Seeds (like black sesame, pumpkin, hemp, cumin, flax)
- Raw cacao butter
- Sea-animal-based omega-3 fatty acids (from wild-caught fish, like salmon)
- Coconut oil as a source of medium-chain triglycerides
- Occasional grass-fed meats or butter from raw grass-fed organic milk

Intermittent Fasting

One of the latest trends is intermittent fasting, based on research that shows links between longevity and caloric restriction. There are various ways to do intermittent fasting—for example, the 5:2 diet, which includes a dramatic restriction on caloric intake for two days a week (down to 500 or 600 calories on each of those days), and the 16:8 diet (also known as the 8-Hour Diet), in which all eating is limited to an eight-hour chunk of time each day, with no caloric intake the other sixteen hours. The goal of these diets is primarily weight loss and longevity, so any benefit for overall health is related to that.

The science behind these diets is based largely on animal studies, which show greater weight loss, a longer lifespan, and fewer diseases in animals made to intermittently fast, *but such outcomes haven't been shown in humans.* What has been shown in humans is that eating fewer calories in general is one of the best proven ways to decrease the impact of aging on the body and brain, so to the extent that intermittent fasting leads to decreased caloric intake, it is likely to benefit longevity. These diets can be very hard to follow. If you try one, the important thing to remember is to keep making healthy choices, no matter how many calories you're eating. Obviously, this type of diet is especially not recommended for anyone with blood sugar issues. They're also not particularly good for those of you looking to gain lean muscle mass. However, it is a fact that a general rise in caloric intake over the last thirty years has accompanied the epidemic of obesity we're seeing, so cutting back on calories, whether through intermittent fasting (which will help lead to a decrease in unhealthy habits like late-night snacking) or simply focusing on decreasing portion sizes, is a helpful way to reduce calories and decrease your risk for preventable causes of death like diabetes, heart disease, and cancer.

Whole-Food Plant-Based Diet

While there have always been vegetarians and vegans, there has been increased attention on whole-foods plant-based diets after the success of the book *The China Study* and the documentary based on this book, *Forks over Knives.*[7] The book focuses on the knowledge gained from a large twenty-year study done in China that looked at correlations between diet, heart disease, and cancer. This study, a joint project of Cornell University, Oxford

University, and the Chinese Academy of Preventive Medicine, showed that high consumption of animal-based foods is associated with more chronic disease, while those who ate primarily a plant-based diet were the healthiest. This study is one of the most respected that has ever been done on human nutrition due to the large size of the sample population and the rigor used in the analysis. The research revealed that such a diet could prevent and even reverse type 2 diabetes and heart disease, and reduce the risk of some forms of cancer. Books such as *The China Study* and other proponents of plant-based diets have popularized the idea of food as medicine by showing that eating right can be as powerful as taking medications for some chronic diseases.

In fact, plant-based diets have been shown in many studies to have advantages in terms of heart disease risk, cancer risk, and diabetes treatment and prevention. For example, the Adventist Health Studies showed that vegetarians had half the risk of developing diabetes as non-vegetarians. A large randomized trial comparing a low-fat vegan diet with a diet following American Diabetes Association guidelines showed that the vegan diet was better in terms of blood sugar and cholesterol control.[8] Overall, says a 2010 report of the U.S. Dietary Guidelines Advisory Committee to the Departments of Agriculture and Health and Human Services, plant-based diets are associated with a reduced risk of cardiovascular disease and mortality.[9]

Personally, I prefer the term "whole-food plant-based diet" to "vegetarian" or "vegan." First of all, the latter terms are generally defined by what they exclude rather than include. Second, "plant-based" emphasizes that fruits are equally important. Third, I believe that a diet doesn't have to be all or nothing, meaning you can transition to eating more plant-based foods without being 100 percent vegetarian or vegan and still experience some of the many health benefits of such an approach to eating.

There is a misconception that eating a plant-based diet precludes improving athletic performance or building muscle mass. In fact, more and more professional athletes have gone plant-based without it harming their athletic performance, including NFL players with plenty of muscle. The list of plant-powered successful athletes is long and includes bodybuilder and Olympian Kendrick Farris, tennis champion Venus Williams, and ultra-Ironman Rich Roll. When my patients point to skinny vegans as evidence of their concern about losing gains made at the gym if they eat more plants and less animal protein, I point to Chicago Bears defensive lineman David Carter, who's 300 pounds of plant-powered muscle.

A plant-based diet doesn't have to exclude all animal products. It can mean substituting plant foods for meat in some meals, such as on "meat-less Mondays." While it is important to be knowledgeable about plant-based sources of amino acids and fats, it is not complicated. Simply make sure you eat a mix of fruits and vegetables, including leafy greens, cruciferous vegetables like broccoli, legumes, nuts, and seeds. If you are eating little or no dairy or other animal products, consider supplementing with vitamins D_3 and B_{12}. Those are the essentials for getting all the nutrients you need on a plant-based diet.

Food Quality (Organics, GMOs) and Impact on Health

What about organics foods and GMOs (genetically modified organisms)? Organic food production avoids the use of pesticides, artificial fertilizers, growth hormones, and antibiotics. Proponents cite evidence that eating organic foods leads to less exposure to toxins, less impact on gut bacteria, and higher nutrient density. In fact, studies do show that organic produce is more nutritious. In a review of over 340 published papers comparing organic and nonorganic foods, organic crops were higher in essential minerals, phytonutrients, and vitamin C and lower in heavy metal and pesticide contamination than nonorganics. Phytonutrients are substances found in plants that help protect plants from germs, fungi, bugs, and other threats—and also are beneficial to human health. It makes sense that fruits and vegetables grown organically contain higher levels of protective substances like antioxidants, since they have to make more of their own protection against damage than do plants that are sprayed with chemicals to protect them.[10]

The research on the health advantages of eating all-organic in terms of toxin exposure is sparser, but it stands to reason that less exposure to toxins is better for our health. The Environmental Working Group (EWG.org) publishes a helpful guide of which types of produce typically have higher levels of pesticide residues—what they call the Dirty Dozen. On the other end of the spectrum, the Clean Fifteen are typically less laden with chemicals, so it may not be worth the extra money to buy these organic (see Box 3.1).

The big questions are about genetically modified crops. In the United States, about 90 percent of corn and soy is GMO. Much of this is used for animal feed, and many corn- and soy-based products are processed and

Box 3.1 Which Produce Should Be Organic

These foods, the "Dirty Dozen," frequently have higher levels of pesticide residues, so it's best to look for organic:

1. Strawberries
2. Spinach
3. Nectarines
4. Apples
5. Grapes
6. Peaches
7. Cherries
8. Pears
9. Tomatoes
10. Celery
11. Potatoes
12. Bell peppers

These foods, the "Clean Fifteen," tend to have lower levels of pesticide residues, so it's okay to buy these conventionally grown:

1. Avocados
2. Sweet corn
3. Pineapples
4. Cabbage
5. Onions
6. Sweet peas, frozen
7. Papayas
8. Asparagus
9. Mangoes
10. Eggplant
11. Honeydew melons
12. Kiwis
13. Cantaloupes
14. Cauliflowers
15. Broccoli

Source: EWG's Guide to Pesticides in Produce

used in everything from sweeteners to protein supplements, so even if we avoid directly eating GMO plant foods, they are present throughout our food supply. Genetic modification is used to make crops more resistant to insecticides and weed-killing chemicals, to help plants tolerate environmental stress, and to make them more appealing to the consumer. Are they safe? The jury is still out.

The one type of GMO crop that we do have data on is Roundup Ready crops such as wheat, corn, and soy. Roundup is the brand name of a weedkiller, glyphosate, made by Monsanto. Farmers use Roundup Ready crops so that they can spray glyphosate on their crops to kill weeds without damaging the crops. While glyphosate itself hasn't been proven to be toxic to human cells, it has been shown to be toxic to our gut bacteria. The damage it causes to gut bacteria impacts our ability to digest food properly and to keep a healthy colonic barrier, as described above. So the concern is that eating food from Roundup Ready crops exposes us to higher levels of glyphosate, negatively impacting the bacteria we need in our colon to keep us healthy. Disturbances in gut bacteria are linked with many issues, from depression to gluten intolerance (ever wonder why suddenly everyone seems to be gluten-sensitive?), irritable bowel syndrome, autism, and many neurological conditions.[11]

Pete's Successful Diet Change

Pete, whom we met in Chapter 2, is our friend with the high risk of heart disease based on his diet, cholesterol, and genes. He tried to eat the low-fat diet recommended by his doctor, but it was a dramatic change, and to him it felt like a punishment—how could he eat out with friends or enjoy going to a BBQ without feeling stressed about his choices? What finally helped was going through an organized four-month lifestyle-change program along with other men and women who had high cholesterol or who had had a recent heart attack. Many medical centers and even some health plans sponsor such "heart-healthy" groups. The program included weekly exercise, some meditation, group discussion and support, and assistance in implementing a low-fat, mostly plant-based diet. He felt like he couldn't have made the dietary change without the weekly meetings, where he had the chance to talk with others trying the same changes, and meetings with a nutritionist to help him plan his meals around his life instead of just giving him a list of dos and don'ts. As a result of making these changes, Pete had a follow-up scan showing regression of the plaque in his arteries, lost fifteen pounds, and felt better than he had in years.

Jim's Ketogenic Diet

Jim is a fifty-five-year-old patient of mine who was noticing some forgetfulness and difficulty with mental focus. His mother had developed Alzheimer's in her sixties, and while he hadn't had any genetic testing, he was convinced he had an inherited predisposition to dementia. He was otherwise generally healthy, with no sign of high blood pressure, overly high cholesterol, or any history of heart disease. I recommended he try eating a more ketogenic-style diet, especially limiting gluten and refined grains. Jim felt he was improving gradually, but his wife said she noticed a difference within a month—she could tell Jim was less likely to forget things or lose his train of thought. Jim might eventually start medication to help slow any progression of mild dementia, but meanwhile, the ketogenic diet is doing the trick.

The Bottom Line

While the nutritional lever is a crucial one for optimal health, there is not one right diet for everyone. The right diet for you depends on your goals and your individual risks for health problems based on your health history, genes, and current lifestyle. In this chapter, I've provided some basic information on common healthy diets currently being promoted and what types of risks each can help to counter. If it all seems overwhelming, remember they all have in common the following:

- Minimize your consumption of processed foods. Eat foods that are as similar as possible to how they are found in nature.
- Minimize your intake of sugars—that includes sodas and juices.
- Eat more plant-based foods: whole fruits, vegetables, nuts, seeds, beans.
- When eating animal products, choose wild, organic, and grass-fed.
- Limit your consumption of saturated animal fats.
- Control your portion size and calorie intake.

You can't go wrong with the general anti-inflammatory diet and more of a plant-based diet. Most experts quote health journalist and writer Michael Pollan, who in his bestselling book *Omnivore's Dilemma* sums up his recommendations for the healthiest diet based on extensive research as: "Eat food. Mostly plants. Not too much."

If you're still not sure what is best for you, ask your doctor to help you identify the most pressing health risks in your own life and which diet type is most likely to prevent problems down the road.

Notes

1. D. Mozaffarian et al., "Changes in Diet and Lifestyle and Long-Term Weight Gain in Women and Men," *New England Journal of Medicine* 364, no. 25 (2011): 2392–2404, doi: 10.1056/NEJMoa1014296.
2. F. B. Hu and W. C. Willett, "Optimal Diets for Prevention of Coronary Heart Disease," *Journal of the American Medical Association* 288 (2002): 2569–2578.
3. Hebrew University of Jerusalem, "Secrets of the Paleo Diet: Archeological Discovery Reveals Plant-Based Menu of Prehistoric Humans," ScienceDaily, December 5, 2016, www.sciencedaily.com/releases/2016/12/161205164935.htm.

4. Philip J. Tuso, "Nutritional Update for Physicians: Plant-Based Diets," *Permanente Journal* 17, no. 2 (2013): 61–66, doi: 10.7812/TPP/12-085. This is an excellent summary of the advantages of a plant-based diet and includes data on the health consequences of relying on a diet with too much emphasis on animal protein.

5. National Health Service of the United Kingdom's Top Diets Review found at https://www.nhs.uk/live-well/healthy-weight/top-diets-review

6. D. Ornish et al., "Intensive Lifestyle Changes for Reversal of Coronary Heart Disease," *Journal of the American Medical Association* 280, no. 23 (1998): 2001–2007. Doi:10.1001/jama.280.23.2001

7. T. Colin Campbell and Thomas M. Campbell II, *The China Study: The Most Comprehensive Study of Nutrition Ever Conducted and the Startling Implications for Diet, Weight Loss, and Long-Term Health* (Dallas, TX: BenBella Books, 2016).

8. Neal D. Barnard et al., "A Low-Fat Vegan Diet and a Conventional Diabetes Diet in the Treatment of Type 2 diabetes: A Randomized, Controlled, 74-wk Clinical Trial," *American Journal of Clinical Nutrition* 89, no. 5 (2009): 1588S–1596S, doi:10.3945/ajcn.2009.26736H.

9. *Report of the Dietary Guidelines Advisory Committee on the Dietary Guidelines for Americans, 2010* (Washington, DC: Agriculture Research Service, US Department of Agriculture, US Department of Health and Human Services, 2010).

10. M. Baranski et al., "Higher Antioxidant and Lower Cadmium Concentrations and Lower Incidence of Pesticide Residues in Organically Grown Crops: A Systematic Literature Review and Meta-analyses," *British Journal of Nutrition* 112, no. 5 (2014): 794–811, doi: 10.1017/S0007114514001366. The idea that more stress on plants makes them healthier (xenohormesis) is akin to the idea of intermittent fasting making humans healthier. This topic has been written about by Michael Gregor of the American College of Lifestyle Medicine on the website NutritionFacts.org. I will have more on this concept as it applies to fitness and recovery in Chapter 13.

11. A. Samesel and S. Seneff, "Glyphosate, Pathways to Modern Diseases II: Celiac Sprue and Gluten Intolerance," *Interdisciplinary Toxicology* 6, no. 4 (2013): 159–184, doi: 10.2478/intox-2013-0026. This review article from researchers at MIT goes into detail, in a way that is understandable, about the proven links between glyphosate and numerous human diseases. The gut-brain connection is laid out beautifully in David Perlmutter with Kristin Loberg, *Grain Brain: The Surprising Truth About Wheat, Carbs, and Sugar—Your Brain's Silent Killers* (New York: Little, Brown, 2013), which also goes into detail on the connection between glyphosate, the health of the gut, and neurological disorders. More about this in Chapter 12, on brain aging.

Resources

For further information on the general diets described in this chapter, see these resources:

Overall: NutritionFacts.org is a great collection of continuously updated scientific articles and videos related to nutrition. It favors plant-based diets but is an excellent general resource.

Paleo: One of the veteran promoters of paleo is Rob Wolf, and while I don't support a strict paleo approach for the reasons mentioned in this chapter, his site, RobWolf.com, does include useful resources about the paleo approach and how it compares to other diets.

Low-carb/ketogenic: Dr. David Perlmutter, an integrative neurologist, has excellent resources on the ketogenic diet on his site, DrPerlmutter. com, especially as it pertains to brain health. His book *Grain Brain* lays out the evidence for the connection between gluten and neurological problems.

Low-fat: Dr. Dean Ornish's lifestyle change program is a proven model for reversal of heart disease. The nutrition section on his site, https:// www.ornish.com/undo-it, has useful tips for a heart-healthy low-fat diet. While insurance usually covers the Ornish program, there may be others available where you live that are similar and less expensive.

Plant-based: As mentioned, the movie *Forks over Knives*, based on the book *The China Study* about the health benefits of a plant-based diet, has spawned a real movement. The website https://www.forksoverknives. com has excellent resources, tips, and links.

Intermittent fasting: The book *The 8-Hour Diet* by former *Men's Health* editor Dave Zinczenko lays out the most popular version of the intermittent fasting approach. I don't agree with his recommendations to eat pretty much anything you want in those eight hours, but this is a good resource to start with when researching this diet.

4

What Supplements to Take for Optimal Health

o you need to take a bunch of supplements on top of eating right? I include supplements within the nutrition lever, because they are useful tools to, as their name says, supplement your diet in order to make sure you are optimizing the raw materials your body needs to stay as healthy as possible for as long as possible. The truth is, most guys could use a little help getting all they need, and many supplements can help with specific issues. Whether you want to improve your performance at the office, at the gym, or in the bedroom, supplements can give you the boost you need to be your most vital self.

The use of herbal supplements has increased dramatically over the past thirty years. Dietary supplements are used by most Americans, with some surveys indicating use by up to 70 percent of the population.[1] Men are big purchasers of supplements, especially for athletic performance (over 80 percent of athletes take three or more supplements), prostate health (over 70 percent of men with prostate cancer take supplements), and sexual performance. But there are some things to know about supplements in the United States before going out and purchasing a bunch.

Dietary supplements are classified as such by the U.S. Dietary Supplement Health and Education Act (DSHEA) of 1994 and are not regulated by the FDA. That means herbal supplements—unlike prescription drugs—can be sold without being tested to prove they are safe and effective. And quality is variable. In 2015 a report came out showing that the *majority* of supplements from large, national retailers don't contain what they claim on the label.[2] Supplement companies often put a seal or stamp on their website or product labels with words such as "Certified GMP," "FDA Approved Facility," or "CGMP Inspected Facility." In truth, there is no "official" seal or stamp, and use of the FDA's logo is misleading, since the FDA does not approve or certify facilities or dietary supplement products. It is true that companies must comply with CGMP (certified good manufacturing practices) regulations. What does that mean? Just that the corporation performs its own lab inspection to verify that the product contains no contaminants (microbes, metals), that the labeling is accurate, and that the supplement can effectively be released into the body. But the manufacturers themselves are responsible for ensuring that the dietary supplement product they introduce into the market is safe.

The issue of adulteration and contamination is also a concern. Men are the primary consumers of two of the three categories of products that are most commonly adulterated in the marketplace: bodybuilding and sexual enhancement agents. The third category is weight loss supplements. Studies have shown that anywhere from 10 to 70 percent of weight loss supplements include pharmaceutical products not listed on the label.

But don't throw the baby out with the bathwater. There are good-quality supplements out there that can have a meaningful and beneficial impact on your health, helping you to achieve your goals. One way to verify the quality of a supplement is to see if it is labeled "USP"—this stands for United States Pharmacopeia and is a marker of that supplement having passed rigorous quality measures. The problem with becoming USP-certified is that it is an expensive process for the manufacturer, and few supplement companies use it. Still, if you see the USP seal, you can feel fairly certain that the product is a good-quality one. Another certification body is NSF International, which verifies the purity of some supplements.

Two excellent resources are ConsumerLab.com and the Natural Medicines Comprehensive Database, which evaluates many different nutritional and herbal supplements for quality, safety, and efficacy. Unfortunately, the use of these databases requires a subscription.

Lastly, it is important to consider interactions between dietary supplements and any medications you may be taking. This is an underappreciated risk but a real one, especially for men on blood thinners such as Coumadin (warfarin), Xarelto (rivaroxaban), or Plavix (clopidogrel). For all of these reasons, it is important to discuss with your practitioner any supplements you are considering taking. If he or she isn't sure about quality brands or drug interactions, seek help from a provider who has experience with supplements.

What to Look for in Supplements

- Check for USP mark or NSF certification, verifying high quality.
- Check a particular brand's quality on ConsumerLab.com.
- Check your choices with a medical professional to help verify quality and possible interactions with medications or other supplements.

There will be more detail on supplements for particular issues in the following chapters that focus on specific conditions. Aside from these specific health concerns, there are some general supplements that might be worthwhile to consider, depending on your own specific goals and issues, so, beyond the specific supplements for particular conditions, here is my top-ten list of dietary supplements for men.

1. Multivitamins

There are so many mixed reports on the value of multivitamins. Most studies showing no impact have used poor-quality multis, so it is hard to say whether or not a good-quality, food-based multivitamin is important to take. Generally, it is always better to get nutrients the way nature made them—in food. But if you don't eat plenty of fruits and vegetables (at least five servings a day), it is probably a good idea to take a high-quality multivitamin. There are a few caveats, though. Look for a multivitamin without iron, as that is not needed by most men. Also look for one without excessive calcium (no more than 500 mg), as there is some evidence of a link between calcium supplementation and increased prostate cancer risk. This will be discussed in greater detail in Chapter 10, on cancer prevention.

2. Fish Oil

After a good multivitamin, my next recommendation is almost always a supplement that contains the omega-3-fatty acids EPA and DHA (eicosapentaenoic acid and docosahexaenoic acid). These fatty acids are some of the most important compounds our bodies use in the fight against disease and inflammation—they have been shown to help lower cholesterol and decrease inflammation in general. Fish oil, which is a good source of both of these, can help prevent and treat heart disease, particularly if you've already experienced a cardiac event, and it helps with depression and ADHD (attention deficit hyperactivity disorder).[3]

Most of us get way too much omega-6 fatty acids, which can be inflammatory, in our food. So it is essential to balance the ratio of omega-6 to omega-3 fatty acids in our body by supplementing with omega-3s alone. Fish oil is the best source, but vegans can use algae-based omega-3 or flaxseed oil. Flaxseed includes a different form of omega-3 fatty acids that is beneficial but generally less potent. Some people do report uncomfortable burping that tastes like fish with certain forms of fish oil, but if you notice that issue, that doesn't mean you'd experience it with other brands. Try another formulation if you need to—it's worth finding a brand that works for you and your body.

3. Vitamin D

This vitamin, which commonly is low in men, is so important because it affects so many of our systems. Vitamin D is actually a hormone, impacting our immune and neurological function, and especially our bone and cardiovascular health. It is produced in the skin from sun exposure and found in fatty fish, cheese, egg yolks, and foods fortified with vitamin D such as dairy, soy milk, and orange juice. Low vitamin D is associated with multiple sclerosis and pain conditions. The amount you take should be chosen to keep your blood levels of 1,25-hydroxy-vitamin D between 50 and 100 ng/ml. Look for cholecalciferol (vitamin D_3) as opposed to ergocalciferol (vitamin D_2), as D_3 is much better absorbed. It is difficult to find vegan forms of D_3 but not impossible. It is important to monitor your blood levels if you are supplementing, because excessively high levels can be dangerous.

4. Vitamin B_{12}

Vitamin B_{12} deficiency (blood levels under 150 μmol/L) is associated with cognitive impairment. The best sources for B_{12} include eggs, dairy products, meat, fish, and fortified soy products. A review of forty-three studies found that vitamin B_{12} levels in the low normal range (<150-250 μmol/L) are associated with Alzheimer's disease, vascular dementia, and Parkinson's disease. As the incidence of type 2 diabetes is increasing exponentially, more and more people are being placed on metformin, a drug shown in multiple studies to deplete vitamin B_{12} levels. You should ask for a check of your vitamin B_{12} status if you are over the age of sixty-five, following a vegan diet, taking metformin or proton pump inhibitors (acid blockers), and/or having signs of cognitive impairment.[4] You can take too much B_{12}, though, so do have your level checked if you are supplementing.

5. Magnesium

Magnesium is particularly important in men's health given its impact on cardiovascular disease and diabetes as well as its role in muscle pain. Magnesium is required in cells to make protein and replicate DNA, as a cofactor for enzymes, and to play important roles in neuromuscular transmission and the regulation of insulin. About 60 percent of adults in the United States do not get enough magnesium, and research shows that a deficiency of this mineral may contribute to atherosclerosis, hypertension, osteoporosis, diabetes mellitus, and higher risk of cancer of the colon and pancreas. In fact, low serum magnesium levels are associated with higher mortality in general, possibly due to such cancers or an increased risk of left ventricular hypertrophy (enlargement of the heart) when magnesium levels are chronically low. The best way to monitor levels is through a red blood cell (rbc) magnesium level, as opposed to a regular serum magnesium level. People on proton pump inhibitors such as Pepcid (famotidine) and Nexium (esomeprazole) are especially at risk for deficiency. Magnesium supplementation has been shown to help blood pressure and insulin sensitivity, and because magnesium is a muscle relaxant, supplementation can reduce muscle strain. Lastly, magnesium can help with sleep—try taking 500 mg of magnesium gluconate at bedtime or 400 mg of liquid ionic magnesium. If it makes your stools loose, you can take a combination of calcium (which counters the stool-softening effects of magnesium) and magnesium, but keep the calcium at 500 mg or below.[5] Magnesium is naturally found in beans and nuts, pumpkin seeds, leafy greens, and whole grains.

Which Form of Magnesium Should You Take?

Magnesium comes in many forms. The best-absorbed is magnesium gluconate. There's some exciting data about magnesium threonate possibly contributing to improved learning and memory, but it's not clear how well it's absorbed. Magnesium citrate is the most common but can cause loose stools. Magnesium sulfate is used as Epsom salts in the bath to relax muscles and ease aches and pains. Liquid ionic magnesium is a form that especially helps with overall relaxation and rest, so it's great for bedtime use.

6. Zinc

Zinc is important for growth, sexual maturation, and reproduction in men. Zinc concentrations are very high in the male genital organs, particularly in the prostate gland, which is largely responsible for the high zinc content in semen. Sperm themselves also contain zinc. Zinc deficiency leads to hypogonadism and infertility in men. One study found improved fertility in men given zinc supplements, including a 74 percent increase in normal sperm count in subfertile men after supplementation of zinc given along with folic acid.[6] Zinc, at doses of 30 mg per day, has also been shown to be beneficial in acne. When zinc is taken at doses of 30 mg per day or higher, 1–2 mg of copper should be taken simultaneously to prevent deficiency, as the two minerals work together. Zinc is plentiful in pumpkin seeds, meat, spinach, cashews, mushrooms, and chickpeas.

7. Coenzyme Q10

Coenzyme Q10, sometimes called CoQ10, works as a preventative for heart health. It's an essential enzyme, but studies show those who are affected by heart disease and cancer are typically low in CoQ10. CoQ10 is important in the formation of ATP (packets of energy) in the mitochondria, so without CoQ10, energy production suffers. It is naturally found in meat as well as spinach, broccoli, and cauliflower. CoQ10 is especially important for men taking statin drugs for cholesterol, as it reduces the muscle pain side effects of statins by countering the damage to mitochondria these pharmaceuticals can cause. I recommend 100 mg of CoQ10 to nearly everyone on a statin drug.

8. Adaptogens: Ashwagandha, Maca, and Ginseng

These are all male energy enhancers, considered adaptogens because they help us deal with biological, mental, and environmental stress and improve vitality. It is not coincidence that every culture seems to have some herb that helps improve male energy. None of these increase testosterone levels per se, but they exhibit many of the effects we traditionally ascribe only to that all-important male hormone. Ashwagandha has long been used in Ayurveda, a medical tradition that comes from India and is perhaps the world's oldest holistic system. Ashwagandha has been shown to help adrenal and thyroid gland function, reduce anxiety and depression, increase stamina and strength, and improve energy in general. A recent study showed that ashwagandha improved muscle strength and recovery in men performing resistance training, including those with little experience working out. It is sometimes considered the "Indian ginseng," but in fact it has as much or more impact than the true ginsengs.[7]

Maca, sometimes called "Peruvian ginseng," has traditionally been used by certain Native American groups in South America. It is a root, looking something like a giant radish, that grows in the Andes. Some studies show it boosts sexual well-being; a particularly well-respected double-blind randomized controlled trial showed that at a dose of 3 g a day, maca reversed many of the sexual side effects experienced by people taking SSRI-medications like Prozac (fluoxetine) for depression.[8]

While several species of ginsengs have been used by traditional Chinese medicine, the form most proven to help male energy and libido is *Panax ginseng* (also called Asian or Korean ginseng). Other ginsengs are American ginseng (*Panax quinquefolius*) and Siberian ginseng (*Eleutherococcus senticosus*, which is not a true ginseng at all; it is more useful for immune function enhancement than as an adaptogen).

I don't recommend taking all three of these adaptogenic herbs, but you can try one at a time to see if you notice a difference in how you feel after using each for a month or so. The ginsengs have quite a few drug-herb interactions, so check with your doctor before starting if you take any prescription medications.

9. L-Theanine

This amino acid, naturally found in tea, can simultaneously reduce anxiety and increase cognitive function, enabling a state of relaxed concentration. It helps boost feel-good neurotransmitters like GABA and dopamine and may even improve libido. Theanine can improve focus and even test performance without the agitation caused by caffeine. It is great to take at night, at a dose of 100 mg, when anxious thoughts inhibit relaxation.

10. Schisandra

Schisandra is an underutilized natural botanical from traditional Chinese medicine that has many benefits for men, including helping with resistance to disease; reducing anxiety; increasing energy and physical performance; and improving sleep, digestion, liver function, adrenal function, and even mental stamina and sexual function. I tend to be skeptical of anything that touts this many benefits, but there are good studies backing all of these up, mostly from China, where this medicinal berry grows.[9] There are few adverse side effects or drug-herb interactions, but be cautious if you take blood thinners or have had an organ transplant, as it can increase metabolism of drugs in the liver, resulting in a decreased amount of drug in the bloodstream. You can take schisandra as a tea, as a tincture, or in capsules of about 500 mg.

Pete's Supplement Regimen

Our friend Pete, with the high risk of heart disease, is eating well and exercising, but also wanted to know if he should take supplements to help his weight, cholesterol, or blood sugar. He is on a statin drug for his cholesterol, so I definitely recommended he take 100 mg of coenzyme Q10. He should also take omega-3 fatty acids (as fish oil) to provide a total of 2,000 mg of EPA and DHA combined , to further help his cholesterol as well as optimize his brain function. I also recommended 400 mg of magnesium gluconate at night to help his heart, 1,000 IU of vitamin D_3 a day, and 1,000 mcg of vitamin B_{12} a day, since he is eating fewer animal products. He can take all these together in the morning with food, except for the magnesium, which he should take at night, as it might help with overall relaxation and sleep.

The Bottom Line

There are many more supplements that are beneficial and much more that can be said about nutrition, but these two chapters on nutrition and supplements were meant to give you a sense of the ways you can use these levers to get you closer to optimal health. As with diet, there is no single best supplement for everyone, so I encourage you to consider your goals and, in consultation with your healthcare practitioner, choose a supplement plan that you can stick with.

Questions to Ask Your Doctor

1. Are there any supplements you think I should be taking?
2. Are there any vitamin or mineral levels you think should be tested given my medical issues and diet? (I would especially recommend having your vitamin D level checked.)
3. Which brands do you recommend for the supplements I should take?

Notes

1. B. B. Timbo et al., "Dietary Supplements in a National Survey: Prevalence of Use and Reports of Adverse Events," *Journal of the American Dietetic Association* 106, no. 12 (2006): 1966–1974.

2. Truman Lewis, "GNC, Target, Walmart, Walgreens Selling Bogus Herbal Supplements, NY Charges," Consumer Affairs, February 3, 2015, https://www.consumeraffairs.com/news/gnc-target-walmart-walgreens-selling-bogus-herbal-supplements-ny-charges-020315.html.

3. D. Mozaffarian and J. H. Wu, "Omega-3 Fatty Acids and Cardiovascular Disease: Effects on Risk Factors, Molecular Pathways, and Clinical Events," *Journal of the American College of Cardiology* 58, no. 20 (2011): 2047–2067, doi: 10.1016/j.jacc.2011.06.063.

4. E. Moore et al., "Cognitive Impairment and Vitamin B_{12}: A Review," *International Psychogeriatrics* 24, no. 4 (2012): 541–556, doi: 10.1017/S1041610211002511.

5. T. Reffelmann et al., "Low Serum Magnesium Concentrations Predict Cardiovascular and All-Cause Mortality," *Atherosclerosis* 219, no. 1 (2011): 280–284, doi: 10.1016/j.atherosclerosis.2011.05.038.

6. W. Y. Wong et al., "Effects of Folic Acid and Zinc Sulfate on Male Factor Subfertility: A Double-Blind, Randomized, Placebo-Controlled Trial," *Fertility and Sterility* 77, no. 3 (2002): 491–498.

7. S. Wankhede et al., "Examining the Effect of *Withania somnifera* (Ashwagandha) Supplementation on Muscle Strength and Recovery: A Randomized Controlled Trial," *Journal of the International Society of Sports Nutrition* 12 (2015): 43, doi: 10.1186/s12970-015-0104-9.

8. C. M. Dording et al., "A Double-Blind, Randomized, Pilot Dose-Finding Study of Maca Root (*L. meyenii*) for the Management of SSRI-Induced Sexual Dysfunction," *CNS Neuroscience and Therapeutics* 14, no. 3 (2008): 182–191.

9. A. Szopa, R. Ekiert, and H. Ekiert, "Current Knowledge of *Schisandra chinenis* (Turcz.) Baill. (Chinese Magnolia Vine) as a Medicinal Plant Species: A Review on the Bioactive Components, Pharmacological Properties, Analytical and Biotechnological Studies," *Phytochemistry Reviews* 16, no. 2 (2017): 195–218.

5

How to Behave for Optimal Health

Two of the powerful levers you can use on your way to optimizing your health are behavior and physical activity. What do those really mean? How can you use these levers to your advantage? This chapter will give you specific ways you can use these tools to work for you and your goals. I will dig deeper into exercise and related supplements in Chapter 13, but because physical activity is one of the most important behaviors for optimal health, I also include it here.

Behavioral Effects on Health

As discussed in Chapter 1, men tend to die before women, statistically speaking, and some of this has to do with their behavior. Men are more likely to overconsume alcohol, smoke cigarettes, and engage in truly risky endeavors. It may be a caricature to say that the typical guy would jump off a roof into a swimming pool or drink excessively before getting behind the wheel of a car more commonly than a woman would, but evidence actually supports this generalization.

Men are more likely to be the victims of auto accidents than women; in fact, men are three times as likely as women to be involved in fatal car accidents. This may be partly due to men being responsible for four out of five DUIs (driving under the influence), but it is also because men are less likely to wear seatbelts and more likely to run yellow lights. Looking beyond motor vehicles, men are more likely to be involved in drug overdoses than women. Studies have found men to underestimate risk and overestimate potential enjoyment from risky behaviors.[1] While there is actually evidence that the difference in risk-taking between genders is narrowing—more and more women are also engaging in risky behaviors that can affect health— men still lead the way.

Alcohol Consumption and Rest

Behaviors such as overconsuming alcohol and getting inadequate rest have large influences on health. Most men can safely consume one to two servings of alcohol a day. What does that mean? Alcohol has similar impacts on health whether it's in beer, wine, or spirits. One serving could be a 12-ounce bottle of beer, a 6-ounce glass of wine, or a 1½-ounce shot of liquor. Actually, unless there's a history of liver problems or addiction, alcohol has a beneficial effect on mortality, with men who have one to two drinks a day having lower mortality than those who don't imbibe at all. But drinking much more than that increases the risk of death.[2] The reduction in risk may be because moderate alcohol consumption lowers the risk of heart disease by increasing HDL (high-density lipoproteins, or "good" cholesterol) and decreasing platelet aggregation (somewhat like the effect aspirin has). Wine seems to have the greatest protective effect, perhaps because it is high in resveratrol, a powerful antioxidant. While it had been thought that red wines exerted a stronger protective effect because of higher polyphenol content, the In Vino Veritas study (Latin for "In wine, truth") showed that the improvement in mortality from alcohol was the same for white wine as for red wine and occurs only among men who exercise.[3] It is not clear why that is the case (perhaps because they didn't burn off the excess calories from the wine?), but those who didn't exercise did not show the same benefits from one to two glasses of wine a day.

As for sleep, this is an underappreciated influence on health. Sleep deficit builds up over time when someone gets less than adequate sleep for many nights in a row. Generally, most adults need seven to nine hours of sleep per night to avoid building up a sleep deficit. Arianna Huffington, journalist and founder of the *Huffington Post*, investigated the effects of sleep deprivation in her book *The Sleep Revolution* and describes how inadequate sleep affects you physically, emotionally, and even financially. Getting less than sufficient sleep contributes to obesity, too. One study showed that men who were limited to only five hours of sleep a night for a week gained an average of two pounds.[4] That may not sound like a lot, but week after week it adds up. It is thought that sleeping less contributes to fatigue, so people who are sleep-deprived eat more to try to get the energy they need to continue functioning. Also, getting less sleep increases the body's production of ghrelin, the hunger hormone, which makes you crave fatty and sugary foods. Sleep deficits have been found to contribute to immune system suppression and, of course, motor vehicle and work accidents. Furthermore, cognitive function gets impaired, we are more likely to overreact, and we are more likely to suffer from depression when we don't get enough sleep. In fact, inadequate sleep is associated with higher risk of death from heart disease and greater mortality overall.[5]

How do you know if you have a sleep deficit? Here's a list of signs that *might* be related to being sleep-deprived.

Symptoms of Sleep Deprivation

1. Gaining weight
2. Being more "on edge" or reactive
3. Having memory issues
4. Having difficulty making decisions
5. Having exaggerated shifts in mood
6. Tripping or difficulty with motor skills
7. Getting sick more easily
8. Falling asleep behind the wheel or during meetings
9. Falling asleep as soon as your head hits the pillow

I recommend using a wearable sleep tracking device if possible. There are many devices available that track activity and sleep, such as the Apple Watch, the Oura Ring, and some of the Garmin sport watches. For me, being able to monitor the quality and length of my sleep gives me insight into the impact of using caffeine, alcohol, or digital devices late at night.

If falling asleep during the day is a problem for you and you snore at night, you should be checked for sleep apnea. This is a common cause of sleep issues, especially among overweight men. Sleep apnea means you actually stop breathing periodically during the night. This can be dangerous, increasing risk for heart attack and stroke. There are ways to treat sleep apnea using appliances like mouth guards and CPAP machines, so it is important to be evaluated by a sleep expert if there is any suspicion that you suffer from this condition.

What about sleeping pills? Many prescription medications like Ambien (zolpidem), Lunesta (eszopiclone), and the benzodiazepines such as Xanax (alprazolam), Klonopin (clonazepam), Ativan (lorazepam), and Valium (diazepam) can help, but they are best used as temporary fixes for occasional difficulties falling asleep. Medications contribute to lesser-quality sleep and can cause side effects and addiction. For example, many people have amnesia or other side effects from zolpidem, and the benzodiazepines are all habit-forming. There are safer natural sleep aids, such as relaxation techniques (meditation or progressive muscle relaxation) or supplements such as melatonin, L-theanine, or valerian root. I recommend trying melatonin first, at a dose of 2–5 mg. Melatonin is a natural hormone that is highest at night. It helps direct your natural circadian rhythm to know when to sleep, so taking melatonin can especially help with jet lag or for people who work long or late hours. Taking it at bedtime helps your brain realize it's time for sleep.

If that doesn't work or if you feel hung over in the morning, I recommend theanine with Relora (an extract of magnolia and Amur cork tree) for anyone who is a little too wired at night to fall asleep. This combination can help to boost the brain's production of the natural relaxing neurotransmitter GABA. Another combination product that works well and is thought to also increase GABA activity includes valerian root, lemon balm, and hops. I will add that CBD (cannabidiol) with or without THC (tetrahydrocannabinol), both from marijuana, has been shown to help with relaxation and with sleep. Of course marijuana is legal in some states and not others. But CBD without THC is legal everywhere and available online. As mentioned in Chapter 4, most supplements are not regulated, so buyer beware. Look for an actual cannabidiol content listed—you'll want at least 30 mg of CBD to see an effect, up to 300 mg. (Some products list the CBD content as a percentage, so you'll need to calculate the number of milligrams based on the concentration and the amount being used.) Of course, check with your doctor before starting any new supplements and especially if you have any chronic medical conditions or take prescription medications, as these supplements can interact with other supplements or medications.

The relaxation techniques I mentioned, such as meditation, are covered in depth in Chapter 6. There are meditation apps and classes in such approaches that make it very easy to try.

Lastly, if you have trouble falling asleep, try turning off all electronics at least an hour before bed. The stimulating effect of the blue light from many devices has been shown to decrease melatonin, increase the amount of time it takes to fall asleep, reduce the amount of REM sleep you get and delay its onset, and reduce alertness in the morning.[6] If you simply cannot avoid screen time in the last hour before bed, at least consider using glasses that filter out the blue light from these devices. It's the blue light that interferes with the brain's ability to enter relaxation mode.

Niko: Sleep Problems

Niko was a fifty-two-year-old patient of mine who told me he had lifelong issues with sleep. He would have some trouble falling asleep and would also wake up in the middle of the night and then have trouble getting back to sleep. Niko has taken Ambien (zolpidem) on and off, but found that occasionally he did something like send an email or eat a snack after taking the medication without remembering anything about it, and this bothered him. He has used Xanax, but he worries about taking it if he's had a beer, and he feels it works less well now than when he first started taking it. These medications did help him fall asleep, but he still awoke around 3:30 a.m. and had difficulty getting back to sleep.

I asked if he snored or if his partner had noticed that he seemed to stop breathing periodically in the middle of the night. Neither of these things rang true for him; if they had, I would have suggested he have a sleep study to look for sleep apnea.

Next I had him work on what we call sleep hygiene. We made sure he reserved his bed for sex or sleep only, limiting the amount of time he spent doing work, answering emails, or watching TV from bed. This helped to train his brain that if he was going to bed (and not engaging in sexual activity), then it was sleep time. I also had him throw a T-shirt on top of his DVR and alarm clock to block out the blue light these machines emit, as the wavelength of that light can interfere with deeper sleep rhythms. I asked him to avoid using any backlit screens such as iPads, laptops, or smartphones for at least an hour before bed.

Just doing these things helped him stay asleep longer into the night, but didn't really help him on nights when he couldn't fall asleep. We tried having him take 2.5 mg of melatonin at bedtime, but he felt a little groggy in the morning after taking it. I asked him to download a meditation app that allowed him to listen to a calming voice after he got into bed. He wasn't looking at the device—simply listening to it. The voice talked him through something called progressive muscle relaxation. This means it had him concentrating on tightening and then immediately relaxing every part of his body, going body part by body part, starting with his toes and working his way up the body. This sort of guided meditation forced Niko to be very present and focused on his body and his breathing instead of worrying about falling asleep or whatever was making him anxious. He found he naturally fell asleep before the voice even got to his upper body. More important, because the relaxation technique had decreased the activity of his sympathetic nervous system, he was able to stay asleep a little longer. When we then added 100 mg of L-theanine to his bedtime ritual, he began sleeping through the night and felt more rested in the morning on a more consistent basis than ever before.

Tips for Better Sleep

Cover little blue lights in the bedroom (from your TV, DVR, alarm clock, chargers, etc.).

Use the bed for sex or sleep only.

Turn off backlit devices at least an hour before bedtime.

Do a relaxation practice after getting into bed (visual imagery, meditation, progressive muscle relaxation).

Try aromatherapy with lavender oil.

Exercise and Health

Now let's look at one of the most important behaviors that correlates with better health: physical activity.

In the United States, only 31 percent of men report engaging in regular physical activity, defined as three sessions a week of vigorous activity (really breaking a sweat) or five sessions per week of light to moderate physical activity (walking the dog, walking on a treadmill while reading an article) lasting thirty minutes or more. Although it may seem obvious that physical activity confers many health benefits, there are multiple studies specifically detailing just how beneficial regular exercise is for health, particularly when considering the diseases most prevalent in men, such as heart disease, metabolic syndrome, obesity, and sexual dysfunction. Studies also show that physical activity is beneficial for the brain, improving mood, helping to stave off age-related memory loss, and improving concentration. Box 5.1 lists the benefits of exercise that are most strongly proven in research studies.[7]

Note the first item in the list. Yes, exercise helps you live longer. At all ages, active people have lower mortality rates than inactive people. Even men who start exercising between ages fifty and sixty have a 49 percent lower death rate than men who stay inactive. A Harvard study of 36,500 male graduates showed that sedentary men gained 1.6 years in life expectancy from becoming active.[8] You may have heard that exercise decreases rate of heart attack, diabetes, and stroke, but did you also know that exercise decreases the risk of colon and lung cancer by about 40 percent? It's

BOX 5.1 20 Health Benefits of Exercise

1. Lower risk of early death
2. Lower risk of coronary heart disease
3. Lower risk of stroke
4. Lower risk of high blood pressure
5. Lower risk of high cholesterol
6. Lower risk of type 2 diabetes
7. Lower risk of metabolic syndrome
8. Lower risk of colon cancer
9. Prevention of weight gain
10. Weight loss, particularly when combined with reduced calorie intake
11. Improved cardiorespiratory and muscular fitness
12. Prevention of falls
13. Reduced depression and anxiety
14. Better cognitive function
15. Better functional health (for older adults)
16. Reduced abdominal obesity
17. Lower risk of hip fracture
18. Lower risk of lung cancer
19. Weight maintenance after weight loss
20. Increased bone density[12]

not known how exactly, but it is thought that the lower risk comes through decreased inflammation and enhanced immune function.[9]

Lastly, not only does physical activity decrease the risk of erectile dysfunction (by decreasing the risk of blood flow blockage from plaque, a consequence of losing weight and reducing cholesterol), but a review published in the *Journal of Andrology* that looked at multiple studies noted that exercise was associated with a direct improvement in erectile dysfunction.[10]

Let's say Pete, our friend who has genes that predispose him to heart disease, wants to start an exercise program. What exactly should he do to lower his risks?

The most often studied type of exercise is cardiovascular. This is anything that gets your heart rate up, such as jogging, swimming, cycling, using the elliptical machine, or even walking briskly enough to make you somewhat out of breath.

How much exercise is enough? Most studies compare even moderate amounts to being sedentary, but generally at least three days a week of moderate cardiovascular exercise is best. At least thirty minutes of sustained sweating is needed, in addition to about 10 minutes of warm-up and 10 minutes of cool-down. But high-intensity interval training (HIIT) actually improves weight loss compared to a continuous period of exercising at the same intensity, and it's also has been shown to be better at building endurance and muscle mass. There are different styles of HIIT—some, like Tabata workouts, do twenty seconds of high intensity followed by ten seconds of rest, repeated eight times; others use longer intervals, such as one minute of fast movement followed by two minutes of fairly slow movement. The jury is out on the exact best interval, but I would advise Pete to spend one session a week doing a longer steady-heart-rate workout and one or two weekly interval workouts, perhaps going hard for thirty seconds followed by two minutes of lower-intensity training and repeating that interval five or six times.

One other thing I would note is that in terms of heart attack prevention, exercising regularly has a more powerful effect than taking a statin drug but staying sedentary, as shown by a study of over 10,000 participants through the Department of Veterans Affairs.[11]

Until now I have been speaking of cardiovascular-type physical activity. It is equally important for optimal health to engage in exercise that incorporates resistance, core work, and flexibility.

Resistance training helps build muscle mass and bone health. Plus, the more muscle mass you have, the higher your basal metabolic rate, which means you burn more calories per day. More muscle also contributes to higher testosterone levels, which in turn makes it easier to build even more muscle mass when working out. Resistance training can be done with weights or by using bodyweight, as in yoga, push-ups, and pull-ups.

Core strengthening, such as abdominal exercises and Pilates, can help prevent or treat back pain, because the stronger your core is, the less strain there is on your spine. Stretching can also be accomplished with yoga, and helps with flexibility. It's best to stretch *after* a workout, when the muscles are warmed up, rather than before, when there is a risk of tendon injury. Flexibility is especially important in older people, as increased flexibility is associated with less risk of falls, which can lead to hip fractures and other serious injuries.

Yoga is a great way to work on flexibility, core strength, and some bodyweight training within a single session. Some more vigorous hatha yoga or hot yoga sessions get your heart rate up enough to provide cardio-vascular training as well. So consider yoga as a very efficient way to get all of your exercise needs in.

Ideal Exercise Program for Optimal Health

Sunday: Yoga class, 1 hour

Monday: Rest

Tuesday: 1 hour on an exercise bicycle (10 minutes of warm-up, 40 minutes of high-intensity interval training, and 10 minutes of cool-down), followed by 5 minutes of stretching

Wednesday: Weight circuit training

Thursday: 1 hour of running (indoors or outside, including 10 minutes of warm-up, 40 minutes of interval training, and 10 minutes of cool-down), followed by 5 minutes of stretching

Friday: Yoga class, 1 hour

Saturday: 1 hour of cardio of any type, preferably outside, such as swimming or hiking (including 10 minutes of warm-up and 10 minutes of cool-down), followed by 5 minutes of stretching

I get that it is hard to stay motivated to continue an exercise program. Some people have a health scare that jolts them into becoming active—Pete, for example, whom I've mentioned before, had a scan that showed significant plaque in the arteries around his heart. That was a big wake-up call for him. He quickly got on track with the diet, supplements, and exercise program I was recommending for him.

But Dave, whom we've seen before, felt okay despite being overweight and having high cholesterol, so he needed a different type of motivation to get moving. Dave is a little competitive, so I introduced him to an app and social community called Strava that helped him to catch the exercise bug. Through apps that track his exercise, he can share his workouts and engage in friendly competition with others—competing to see who has the most steps walked, stairs climbed, or minutes run. He can also compare his own performance over time, such as how long it takes him to bike a particular route. There are many apps like this that enable you to share workout information with a chosen social media group, such as coworkers or family members.

For some guys I recommend group exercises. Working out in a group, either in a boot-camp-type class, a CrossFit program, or with a few friends who get together and hire a personal trainer, can be very motivating. The group helps to keep you accountable. A little healthy competition can be just the thing that motivates.

It's important to discuss your plans to start an exercise regimen with your doctor, especially if you are taking medications on a regular basis or dealing with any chronic conditions. Box 5.2 lists other considerations to help you be successful in your fitness endeavor.

The Bottom Line

Move. Staying physically active is one of the most important and most powerful anti-aging things you can do for physical and mental health.

Rest. If you don't sleep enough to feel well rested, follow the sleep tips earlier in this chapter. If you still have problems sleeping through the night, talk to your health practitioner about it. The negative impact of a sleep deficit builds up over time and contributes to significant health problems.

Questions to Ask Your Doctor

1. Am I medically cleared to engage in any exercise program I choose? If you think I have restrictions, what are they?
2. Do I need a stress test before embarking on a new exercise program?
3. Do I need a sleep study? (If you don't feel rested in the morning, ask your doctor about a sleep study or some other way to look into why you are not getting restful sleep.)

Notes

1. Christine Harris and Michael Jenkins, "Gender Differences in Risk Assessment: Why Do Women Take Fewer Risks than Men?," *Judgment and Decision Making* 1, no. 1 (July 2006): 48–63.

2. A. Di Castelnuovo et al., "Alcohol Dosing and Total Mortality in Men and Women: An Updated Meta-analysis of 34 Prospective Studies," *Archives of Internal Medicine* 166, no. 22 (2006): 2437–2445, doi:10.1001/archinte.166.22.2437.

3. M. Taborsky, P. Ostadal, and M. Petrek, "A Pilot Randomized Trial Comparing Long-Term Effects of Red and White Wines on Biomarkers of Atherosclerosis (In Vino Veritas: IVV Trial)," *Bratislavské lekárske listy* 113, no. 3 (2012): 156–158.

4. R. R. Markwald et al., "Impact of Insufficient Sleep on Total Daily Energy Expenditure, Food Intake, and Weight Gain," *Proceedings of the National Academy of Sciences of the United States of America* 110, no. 14 (2013): 5695–5700, doi:10.1073/pnas.1216951110.

5. Arianna Huffington, *The Sleep Revolution: Transforming your Life, One Night at a Time* (New York: Harmony Books, 2016).

6. This study looked at those using a backlit device, such as an iPad, in bed before sleep. The subjects had 55 percent less melatonin production, took an extra ten minutes to fall asleep, and took hours longer to feel alert in the morning. A. Chang et al., "Evening Use of Light-Emitting eReaders Negatively Affects Sleep, Circadian Timing, and Next-Morning Alertness," Proceedings of the National Academy of Sciences 112, no. 4 (2015): 1232–1237, doi: 10.1073/pnas.1418490112.

7. The federal government's Office of Disease Prevention and Health Promotion has excellent resources related to the impact of physical activity on health; see "Physical Activity Has Many Health Benefits," in *2008 Physical Activity Guidelines for Americans*, https://health.gov/paguidelines/guidelines/chapter2.aspx.

8. Liisa Byberg et al., "Total Mortality After Changes in Leisure Time Physical Activity in 50 Year Old Men: 35 Year Follow-up of Population Based Cohort," *BMJ* 338 (2009):b688.

9. I. Thune and A.-S. Furberg, "Physical Activity and Cancer Risk: Dose-Response and Cancer, All Sites and Site-Specific," *Medicine and Science in Sports and Exercise* 33 suppl. (2001): S530–S550. Based on a systematic review of forty-eight studies and over 40,000 cases of the disease, the authors found that physical activity reduces the risk of lung cancer in men by 20–50 percent, with evidence of a dose-response effect.

10. Office of Disease Prevention and Health Promotion, "Physical Activity Has Many Health Benefits."
11. Peter F. Kokkinos et al., "Interactive Effects of Fitness and Statin Treatment on Mortality Risk in Veterans with Dyslipidaemia: A Cohort Study," *Lancet* 381, no. 9864 (2013): 394–399, doi: 10.1016/S0140-6736(12)61426-3.
12. Bruce B. Campbell and Myles D. Spar, "Physical Activity and Men's Health," in *Integrative Men's Health*, edited by Myles D. Spar and George E. Munoz (New York: Oxford University Press, 2014), doi: 10.1093/med/9780199843794.003.0006.

Resources

The Sleep Revolution: Transforming your Life, One Night at a Time by Ariana Huffington (New York: Harmony Books, 2016). In this *New York Times* bestseller Huffington shows how poor sleep compromises our health and our decision-making and undermines our work lives, our personal lives, and even our sex lives.

Tom's Guide to the best fitness trackers: https://www.tomsguide.com/us/best-fitness-trackers,review-2066.html. It can get confusing looking for an exercise or fitness tracker. I like Tom's Guides to all things tech.

6

How to Manage Stress for Optimal Health

Optimal health is about more than excellent physical health; with optimal health, the mind is content and emotions are generally positive. In fact, it has been clearly proven that physical health is influenced by emotional and mental health, so much so that mortality, or risk of death, has been shown to be impacted not only by stress but also by the presence or lack of social connections and by having a sense of purpose. This chapter will explore how the mind interacts with the body and your overall health as well as powerful ways in which emotional, mental, social, and behavioral factors can directly affect health.

For example, we often think that everyone with depression knows they are depressed and feel sad. That's not always the case, especially among men, who may have symptoms that they or their doctor do not recognize as indicators of depression, delaying care and treatment. Men with depression may feel a lack of enjoyment in activities they previously found enjoyable (anhedonia), may feel fatigued, may be eating more than normal or not eating much at all, or may be sleeping excessively or having trouble sleeping.

Symptoms of Depression Among Men

Anhedonia—loss of interest in things that were previously enjoyable

Fatigue—feeling tired all the time

Changes in eating—overeating or loss of appetite

Changes in sleep—sleeping a lot or not sleeping much at all

In fact, mood and anxiety disorders are a common complaint among men. Dan Harris's *New York Times* bestseller *10% Happier* is an excellent description by someone who, despite having panic attacks on live television, was not aware that what he was experiencing was anxiety. Later, however, he discovered the power of a proven mind-body technique to relieve his symptoms.

As Dan writes, the most-proven treatment for anxiety in general and for many other issues is mindfulness-based stress reduction (MBSR). Mindfulness is the nonjudgmental awareness of the present moment. Jon Kabat-Zinn, PhD, a professor at the University of Massachusetts, wrote in his book *Full Catastrophe Living* about learning how to practice mindfulness meditation in an eight-week course that is still taught all over the world.

To sum it up simply, MBSR is about spending some amount of time every day *not* projecting into the future, *not* worrying about the past, and *not* judging oneself or others. The key aspect during meditation sessions is to notice thoughts—not trying to avoid them, but realizing that *you control your thoughts; your thoughts don't control you.*

Why Is Managing Stress So Important?

Stress is the body's natural reaction to crisis, threatening situations, and fear. It is also a good indicator that we are operating at the edge of our comfort zone, an area of growth. This can be positive and important, in that appropriate fear and detection of crisis mean survival, and because growth is what we are all built for. But we are not built for *constant* stress.

The stress response, which involves the adrenal glands and the sympathetic nervous system, is meant for short bursts of activity. With chronic stress, we burn out these systems, resulting in damage to our ability to maintain energy and respond to crises and even causing accelerated aging of the body and brain. In fact, cortisol, the hormone pumped out from the adrenal glands in response to stress, is toxic to brain cells when those cells are exposed to it over extended periods of time.

Cortisol shifts the focus away from activities of rest, relaxation, and repair, such as digesting food, wound healing, and fighting infection. Instead, cortisol dampens our pain response and decreases the inflammatory response in order for us to focus on the task at hand—fighting or fleeing. If we are preparing for battle day in and day out, then our sympathetic nervous system remains on high alert nonstop.

As many as 90 percent of all illnesses have a stress component. Some consequences of a prolonged stress response include cardiovascular disease, recurrent infections, impaired healing, weight gain, insomnia, fatigue (since the body constantly has to be on guard and mobilized), and disruption of memory.

Mindfulness and other forms of meditation elicit what Herbert Benson, MD, of Harvard University's Mind-Body Medical Institute, calls the "relaxation response," which is the polar opposite of the chronic stressed physiology just described. Modern imaging with PET scanning and advanced fMRI technology has shown that meditation actually rewires the brain, creating new pathways in a process called neuroplasticity. The practice of mindfulness has been shown to increase activation of the prefrontal cortex, which is associated with greater adaptive responses to negative or stressful life events and significant reductions in anxiety and negative affect. Scans show that the brain's fight-or-flight center, the amygdala, enlarges in individuals who are constantly stressed, but after an eight-week course of mindfulness practice, it shrinks down to a healthier size.

It should also be mentioned that mindfulness has been shown to operate not only on the brain and hormone levels but also on the genetic level. Yes, mindfulness changes gene expression by decreasing the expression of genes associated with inflammation, the factor behind many diseases of aging. The most exciting thing is that when genetic expression changes, these changes can get passed down to future generations. So your engaging in mindfulness or other mind-body practices can make your future children and grandchildren more resilient and relaxed by nature.

If meditation isn't for you, there are other ways to elicit this same relaxation response, such as journaling, breath work, tai chi, flow yoga (vinyasa), and prayer. Other mind-body techniques include hypnosis, visual imagery, biofeedback, qi gong, cognitive behavioral therapy, group support, spirituality, and even dance. All of these techniques can help with overall relaxation, increased resilience to stress, lowered blood pressure, better moods, higher energy levels, and a more balanced attitude overall. Maybe they sound like they're out of your wheelhouse, but don't rule them out; becoming more in tune with our mind and body is just another tool we can all use toward overall wellness, inside and out, so try one or two of these techniques.

The most important element of any mind-body practice is regular practice. Once a week won't cut it if we're trying to change our brain and decrease our propensity to feel stressed and anxious. Think of mind-body activities like mindfulness as training the brains to be more responsive and less reactive. This takes daily practice, but the benefits are enormous.

An Ideal Week of Daily Mind-Body Practice

Here's a sample week that includes some sort of mind-body practice every day, to keep you more responsive and less reactive.

Sunday: Exercise
Physical activity helps decrease the feeling of stress. A brisk walk can have as much effect as a mild tranquilizer

Monday: Breathe
Ever take a deep breath during a stressful moment and immediately feel more in control? Taking slow, steady, deep breaths activates the parasympathetic nervous system, which is responsible for slowing the heart rate and promoting calm feelings.

Tuesday: Meditate
Try a simple meditation at least one day of the week. There are plenty of apps listed in the resources section of this chapter that can guide you.

Wednesday: Go outside
Spending time outdoors can lower your blood pressure, relax your muscles, and improve your immune system. In Japan, a form of preventive medicine called *shinrin-yoku*, or "forest bathing,"

involves simply walking in the woods. It has been shown to help with mood, focus, and feelings of stress.

Thursday: Visualize

Whether it's the beach, a lush forest, or your bed, mentally visiting a place where you feel safe and content can help calm your nervous system. Spend 5 minutes imagining yourself in such a place. See how relaxed you feel afterward.

Friday: Write

Writing some thoughts about what you are grateful for can change your whole perspective on things—for the better.

Saturday: Rock out

Listening to music you love can calm your nerves. Studies show that from surgeons to presenters in front of an audience, having music on in the background can make you feel less anxious.

Other Mind-Body Influences on Health

Social Connections

Social connections are important for overall health. In fact, lack of social connections cause an increase in mortality on par with smoking fifteen cigarettes a day.[1] Men often have other men to spend time with or watch sports event with, but social connections are about spending time with others with whom you can share thoughts, even the thoughts that make you feel afraid or vulnerable. I have this saying: when men are sad, they are more likely to reach for a beer bottle than a phone. Unfortunately, that reticence to seek out help is a problem for many men. I often encourage patients to seek out group activities around a common interest, to help develop bonds with others who can be sources of support and encouragement.

Having a Purpose

Dan Buettner wrote in his book *The Blue Zones* about the five areas in the world with the longest-living and healthiest populations on earth. The

> # Box 6.1 Attributes Common to the Blue Zones, Where People Live Longer and Healthier than Everywhere Else on Earth
>
> 1. Clear identification of a sense of overall purpose.
> 2. Regular physical activity, such as natural daily movement.
> 3. Active management and reduction of stress.
> 4. The 80 percent rule: stop eating when you're 80 percent full.
> 5. A diet high in plant foods.
> 6. A diet low in meat.
> 7. Having some sort of spiritual practice.
> 8. Caring for and feeling cared for by loved ones.
> 9. Being part of social groups that engage in healthy behaviors.

attributes he identified as common to these areas are listed in Box 6.1. I want to highlight one of the strongest factors that is related to mind-body influence on health—finding one's purpose—because the impact of something as simple as spending time to clearly identify one's sense of purpose is astounding. It turns out that merely having a sense of purpose is associated with a 20 percent decrease in mortality, on par with starting an exercise program and more than quitting smoking. In fact, according to Buettner's book, identifying a clear sense if purpose is associated with adding seven years to life expectancy. Want to add seven years to your life? Spend some time thinking about and clearly articulating what matters *to you*—what your values are, or what you see as the most important reasons to get up every day.

SAM'S STORY

Sam is thirty-eight, with no significant physical problems. But he came in complaining of sleep issues and an inability to lose about ten pounds of excess weight he had been carrying. He was eating well and exercising, but he was stressed about work and not sleeping more than six hours a night, mostly because he had a hard time falling asleep. When we checked Sam's salivary cortisol, we found that his levels of this hormone were constantly higher than normal throughout the day. No wonder he couldn't fall asleep—his stress hormones were telling his body to keep fighting or fleeing, even late at night. If he continued at this rate, his adrenals would burn out, and instead of feeling wired and anxious, he'd be chronically tired and burned out.

I could give Sam a sleeping pill to knock him out, but that wouldn't really get to the cause of his issues. I explained to Sam that some of his weight gain was due to excessive cortisol. Cortisol is similar to prednisone, the steroid people have to take for long periods when they have autoimmune diseases or severe asthma. Ever seen someone on prednisone for a long time? They blow up from retaining salt and water as well as from a ravenous appetite caused by the prednisone. Sam was basically making his own prednisone, in the form of cortisol, all day every day—that was his extra ten pounds.

I recommended supplementing with L-theanine and schisandra to help him relax without making him too drowsy. And I encouraged Sam to try a daily mind-body practice to encourage his adrenal glands to chill out. "It's sort of a fake-it-til-you-make-it approach," I told Sam. "You just have to do some activity like mindfulness, breath work, or journaling *every* day to get your adrenal glands to think everything is under control. If you're spending 20 minutes taking slow, deep breaths, your body will think there is no way you could be in crisis mode, and it will decrease the sympathetic nervous system stress response." Sam decided to try MBSR. He took the eight-week course along with his girlfriend, and it changed his life. After he finished the course he used an app on his smartphone to do a 20-minute mindfulness session at least once a day. It wasn't the 45 minutes that the MBSR teacher suggested, but it was enough to help. Sam realized how much control he had over his own thoughts and learned to build in a half-second pause before reacting to triggers. This made a huge difference in his personal and professional relationships, making his life less stressful all around. After six months, he had lost the ten pounds and was at least 10 percent happier, just as the title of Dan Harris's book predicted.

Mind-Body Approaches and Specific Diseases

Hypertension

In cases of essential hypertension (that is, high blood pressure that doesn't have a known disease-related cause, such as kidney disease or an adrenal tumor), mind-body techniques can be powerful adjuncts to conventional treatment. Breath retraining, biofeedback, and at-home breath pacing devices (such as the Resperate), all of which encourage slow, diaphragmatic breathing, have been shown to reduce systolic blood pressure. Especially when the out-breath is twice as long as the in-breath, slow deep breathing elicits the relaxation response, increases activity of the parasympathetic nervous system (which, unlike the sympathetic nervous system, promotes relaxation), and decreases blood pressure. The ratio of breathing recommended by integrative medicine pioneer Andrew Weil, MD, is 4-7-8: a 4-second inhalation through the nose, 7 seconds of holding the breath, and a slow and steady 8-second exhalation through the mouth. Repeating this cycle four times can help decrease the activity of the sympathetic nervous system, promoting relaxation and sleep.

Stress and the Prostate

Chronically elevated levels of stress hormones have been implicated in the development and worsening of benign prostatic hypertrophy (BPH), a condition common as men age. In BPH the prostate enlarges, causing urinary symptoms such as dribbling, urgency, difficulty with urinary stream, and waking up several times a night to urinate. Furthermore, the stress hormones epinephrine and norepinephrine lead to increased contraction of the pelvic floor as well as the prostate itself, stimulating the need to urinate.

Low Back Pain

Studies have been so definitive about the benefit of mind-body approaches to low back pain that the American College of Physicians (ACP) published guidelines in 2017 for the management of low back pain that included recommendations for MBSR, stating: "For patients with chronic low back pain, ACP recommends that physicians and patients initially select non-drug therapy with exercise, multidisciplinary rehabilitation, acupuncture, mindfulness-based stress reduction, tai chi, yoga, motor control exercise (MCE), progressive relaxation, electromyography biofeedback, low level laser therapy, operant therapy, cognitive behavioral therapy, or spinal manipulation."[2]

Simple Mind-Body Activities You Can Start Right Away

1. Download an app such as Calm, Headspace, or 10% Happier.
2. Try Dr. Weil's 4-7-8 breathing, as described in this chapter.
3. Keep a gratitude journal in which every day you list three to five things you are grateful for.

The Bottom Line

The mind and body are closely linked, with bidirectional influences. While we intuitively know about this link—think of how the heart races when we feel afraid, or how the face blushes when we're embarrassed—the extent of the connection is much more pervasive. Emotions, thoughts, and perceptions are translated chemically and hormonally, affecting our physical health in numerous ways, including cardiovascular health, immune function, sexual function, and even prostate health. There are many proven modalities to help elicit a healthier and more adaptive relaxation response, countering the negative impact of constant stress. Modalities such as mindfulness-based stress reduction and simple breath work can be powerful if used consistently as part of positive lifestyle habits.

Notes

1. Susan Mayor, "Loneliness Is Associated with Higher Risk of Stroke and Heart Disease, Study Finds," *BMJ* 353 (2016): i2269.
2. A. Qaseem et al., "Noninvasive Treatments for Acute, Subacute, and Chronic Low Back Pain: A Clinical Practice Guideline from the American College of Physicians," *Annals of Internal Medicine* 166 (2017): 514–530, doi: 10.7326/M16-2367.

Resources

Further information on mindfulness-based stress reduction: One of the most-researched approaches is MBSR, developed in 1990 by Jon Kabat-Zinn. Group-based MBSR training consists of eight 2½-hour weekly sessions, as well as an additional one-day intensive retreat. Participants are given homework to engage in daily mindfulness exercises and keep track of their experiences, which they share at the following group session. No matter what exercises are practiced during the session or at home, the focus is the same: the cultivation of mindfulness. When yoga postures are introduced during the group session, the emphasis is not on increasing flexibility or strength but on building awareness of the present moment: *How do you feel in your body when you move this way? What thoughts arise as you breathe, twist, turn, stand, or sit? What moods are present right now?* Quickly people confront the realization that most of our lives are spent somewhere other than the present. Instead of feeling the sensations and remaining present to them, most often we judge, evaluate, compare, or try to change. The premise of MBSR is that by learning to embrace the moment without running away from it, we can reduce stress and therefore the subsequent negative physiological, immunological, and psychological impacts. When we learn to cultivate mindfulness, we are, in essence, cultivating our self-regulation capacity. Attending to the moment allows us to become nonreactive self-observers who learn that we are able to choose our mental focus rather than be victim to our thoughts. Learning this mindfulness can increase a sense of agency and self-mastery, where you recognize you do not have to follow every sensation or thought that arises, but merely can witness them like a gentle observer. Remember that you can control your thoughts without having your thoughts control you.

Apps that offer mindfulness guidance:

Headspace: Great for beginners, with a robust free version that includes animations and progress trackers.

Calm: With Calm you can choose the length of your session, from 3 minutes to 25 minutes; receive the Daily Calm, a 10-minute mindfulness session, each day; and get choices of soothing sounds to help with sleep. There's not as much available in the free version, but the paid version is very robust for beginner and experienced meditators alike.

10% Happier: This app is designed for skeptics. It was developed by the author of the book of the same name, Dan Harris, who was a skeptical journalist for ABC news before having an on-air panic attack and delving into the world of mindfulness. This app has a huge variety of mindfulness experiences at all different levels and lengths.

Insight Timer: This app has thousands of free guided meditations. You can't *not* find a background sound, meditation style, or teacher you like if you keep searching on this app.

Stop, Breathe, and Think: This app nicely divides guided meditations into categories, like compassion, depression, anxiety, and sleep.

Websites related to books mentioned:

Dan Harris, 10% Happier: http://www.10percenthappier.com.
Dan Buettner, The Blue Zones: https://www.bluezones.com.

7

How to Minimize Negative Environmental Effects on Optimal Health

Another lever impacting optimal health is the chemical environment in which we live. There is well-founded concern about negative health impacts from the toxins we encounter in our daily lives. While this chapter can't be an exhaustive description of all of the possible environmental toxins that can affect our health, I will focus on those most relevant to men's health: endocrine-disrupting chemicals. These come from pesticides in foods and the air, as well as chemicals we commonly encounter in household cleaners, in skin and hair products, and in everyday plastics. Many plastics, for example, contain phthalates or bisphenol-A (BPA); we find these plastics virtually everywhere, from plastic water bottles to the plastic wrappings on food at the grocery store. These chemicals leach into our food and then, when we eat the food, accumulate in our fat cells, where they can block or mimic normal hormonal actions. Not only can they affect testosterone and estrogen, but they can also affect blood sugar metabolism, increasing risk for metabolic syndrome and diabetes. Pesticides and flame retardants are two other groups of chemicals with significant health effects. Table 7.1 lists some of the symptoms and diseases associated with exposure to these toxins. This chapter will provide more detail about where these chemicals are found, what particular health effects they have, and how you can minimize exposure to them.

Endocrine-disrupting chemicals interfere with the normal functioning of hormones, including sex hormones, the hormones involved in insulin production, and the hormones responsible for bone health.

Studies show that 90 percent of us have traces of BPA in our urine, suggesting we are heavily exposed to it. BPA is used to make hard polycarbonate plastics (those with the recycling code 7 on them), dental sealants, can liners, and thermal paper receipts, among other things. BPA is an estrogenic endocrine disruptor, meaning that it interferes with the action of testosterone. Exposure to BPA is linked with the following conditions:

- Impaired sperm quality
- Heart disease

Table 7.1 Most Common Symptoms and Diseases Influenced by Environmental Chemicals

Symptoms	Diseases
Headaches	Hypertension
Memory loss	Pulmonary fibrosis
Chest pain	Fertility issues
Heart arrhythmias	Sperm issues
Fatigue	Neuropathy
Brain fog, memory issues	Hormone imbalances
Cough, shortness of breath	Prostate cancer
Eczema, other skin conditions	Obesity
Irritable bowel, gastrointestinal disturbances	ADHD
	Allergies
	Asthma
	Thyroid dysfunction

- Diabetes
- Abnormal thyroid function
- Decreased testosterone function[1]

BPA also interferes with glucose metabolism by affecting the enzymes that regulate blood sugar, and it increases overall inflammation in the body by stimulating the release of inflammatory chemicals.

BPA can leach out of plastic most easily when the plastic is heated, so one way to avoid exposure is by making sure you don't heat food in plastic containers or leave BPA-containing water bottles in a hot car. If you do reuse plastic containers, try to avoid those with the recycling code 7 on the bottom (containers with the code 4 are a better choice). For water bottles, choose glass or stainless steel. Because most aluminum cans have BPA in the lining, to decrease your exposure it is best to minimize the consumption of food from cans. It's always a good idea to eat fresh or frozen vegetables anyway, but for canned foods choose glass jars when possible. For beans, consider using dried beans instead of canned.

Phthalates are another category of endocrine-disrupting chemicals. They are used to increase flexibility and durability in plastics, and they are found in food and beverage containers as well as deodorants, insect repellents, air fresheners, laundry detergents, vinyl flooring, shower curtains, raincoats, and even fast food. Phthalates are also found in lubricants, adhesives, wallpaper, cleansers, electronics, and medical tubing. Because phthalates are used in plastic wrap, the chemicals can leach into food wrapped in plastic, especially fatty foods. Phthalates are especially strongly associated with impairment of testosterone and sperm production through their action on androgens. Like with BPA, phthalates have been found in the urine samples of 90 percent of Americans.

Phthalates have been associated with the following conditions:

- Metabolic syndrome (high blood sugar, high blood pressure, and high cholesterol)
- Smaller penis size in babies
- Erectile dysfunction
- Impaired fertility
- Behavioral problems in children

Plastics with phthalates most commonly have the recycling number 3 or 7 on the bottom, so avoiding these and using #4 plastics or glass or stainless steel containers will help decrease exposure. Because phthalates have been found in the water supply, using a home water filtration system can help to limit your exposure as well. I write "home system" as opposed to an in-sink system, because if you want to truly minimize exposure to chemicals, you need to filter the water you bathe in as well. Lastly, look for personal care and cleaning products (deodorants, detergents, colognes, etc.) that are phthalate-free. The Environmental Working Group's website (www. ewg.org) has a list of companies that make such products.

Flame retardants are important in preventing fires but have become so ubiquitous that the chemicals that are used to make them are found in samples of human blood around the world. Unfortunately, they have negative consequences on hormones involved in reproduction and thyroid function as well as overall metabolism, and they can lead to asthma and obesity. Chemicals such as PCBs (polychlorinated biphenyls) and PBDEs (polybrominated diphenyl ethers) are used in many household items, from furniture to computers, to make them flame-retardant, and they make their way into household dust, which is easily inhaled, allowing the PCBs and PBDEs to get into our bloodstream. Also, PCBs from industrial use are often found in lakes and rivers and are therefore commonly found in fish, accumulating in the fatty tissue of people who eat those fish. Nearly everyone in the United States has traces of these chemicals in their bodies. One concern of note for men is that more and more studies are linking PCB exposure to prostate cancer risk.[2]

PDBEs have been largely banned, some since 2004 and others since 2013, but many of the products made before then are still being used. PDBEs especially affect neurological and immune function. It is not known if they impair hormone function.

What can you do to avoid these chemicals? See Box 7.1 for ways to reduce your exposure to PCBs and PDBEs.

Pesticides, such as DDT, and herbicides, like atrazine, impact our endocrine and neurological systems, impacting hormone and neurotransmitter production and function. While DDT is banned in the United States because of its toxicity, it is still being used in the developing world. And other pesticides still in use in the United States are toxic as well. For example, organophosphates are widely used and are known neurotoxins, with occupational exposure being linked to cancer, thyroid disorders, and hyperactivity. The amount found in grains and other foods grown with this specific pesticide has not been associated with human disease, but it has been shown to impact our gut microbiome, and this impact in turn is associated with autoimmune disease, gastrointestinal dysfunction, and allergies. In fact, the International Agency for Research on Cancer, part of the World

Box 7.1 Simple Ways to Reduce Exposure
to Flame-Retardant Chemicals

1. Select carpets, carpet pads, cushions, and upholstered furniture from naturally flame-resistant materials such as wool, polyester, and hemp.
2. Repair rips that expose foam filling, which contains the flame retardants.
3. Clear away dust with a vacuum fitted with a HEPA filter.
4. Wash hands frequently when working around the house.
5. Replace older products containing polyurethane foam, such as televisions, computers, and furniture, with newer ones without PDBEs.

Health Organization, has classified the most commonly used organophosphate, glyphosate (also known as Roundup), as "probably carcinogenic" in humans. This means it would be best to avoid exposure to it by choosing organic grains as much as possible.

Pesticides can act as endocrine disruptors, mimicking estrogen, having anti-testosterone properties, or blocking the action of thyroid hormone. These chemicals also interfere with the function of our mitochondria, the energy-producing parts of all our cells. This mitochondrial toxicity may play a role in numerous diseases such as Parkinson's disease and diabetes. The exact cause is not proven, but there have been many studies showing a link between pesticide exposure and risk of these diseases.

Cellphones give off radio-frequency radiation (RF) (also known as electromagnetic fields or EMF) that has been suspected as contributing to an increased risk of cancer, especially of the head and neck. So far the link has not been proven, but the degree of risk would certainly correspond to the amount of time people are exposed to such radiation and the distance between the source and the body. The American Cancer Society has an excellent summary of the research, which they keep up to date, on their website.[3] But the International Agency for Research on Cancer does classify RF fields as "possibly carcinogenic to humans," so it makes sense to limit the length of use and proximity of cellphones to your body, especially the brain and genital areas.

It is important to note that all of the chemicals mentioned in this chapter as endocrine disrupters or as hormonally active are also considered obesogens (obesity promoters), meaning they disrupt fat metabolism and can cause weight gain. Even worse, many of these toxins are being found to impact gene expression, which means that their effect on hormone activity may be carried down through future generations.

DON'S STORY

Don is a forty-eight-year-old man who recently noticed some decrease in libido. He also told me he had noticed the beginning of "man boobs." Testing showed that his estrogen was normal but his testosterone level was slightly low. It turned out that Don's lunch was usually a frozen entree that he would heat up in the microwave at work. He also kept a case of plastic bottles of water in the trunk of his car. Every day he would take one out and put it in the fridge at work, but the bottles were in his hot car for days on end. Most likely the BPA in the water bottles was leaching into the water, lowering his testosterone somewhat. Also, BPA can attach to estrogen receptors and mimic the role of this hormone, causing an increase in breast tissue. The phthalates in the plastic wrap on his frozen meals also could be contributing to his low testosterone. So I advised him to use a metal water bottle that he could fill up with filtered water, and to heat his meals in a glass or ceramic container. It took several months, but he did notice his "man boobs" shrinking and libido coming back online.

So, what can you do to limit your exposure to all these environmental toxins?

You have to live in the real world, so that means you're sometimes going to use plastic products with these chemicals, you're occasionally going to buy food wrapped in plastic, and you're going to use wireless electronic devices. But here are ten tips to minimize your exposure and therefore decrease your risk of symptoms or diseases associated with chemical exposure.

1. Eat organic. Studies have shown that switching to organics lowers the level of organophosphates and other pesticides in the blood. The Resources section at the end of this chapter directs you to information from the Environmental Working Group about which are the most important fruits and vegetables to buy organic.
2. Check personal care products for parabens (which are estrogenic) and phthalates.
3. Avoid plastics when possible, especially when they have been heated or carry recycling code 3 or 7. Don't drink water from plastic bottles that have been sitting in a hot car for a long time, and don't heat anything up in the microwave in plastic—use glass or ceramic for heating foods and liquids.
4. Try to avoid foods wrapped in plastic, and trim off extra fat from foods that have been wrapped in plastic for any length of time.
5. Use nontoxic cleaning products—look for the words "phthalate-free," especially if the product contains fragrance. Remember that just because a product says "natural," "nontoxic," or "eco-friendly," that doesn't mean it is. Look for a list of ingredients or use a resource like the Environmental Working Group's guide to healthy cleaning (see the Resources section).
6. Avoid furniture with flame retardants. If you see that a piece of furniture contains polyurethane foam or mentions TB-117 (an older technical bulletin requiring certain flame retardants), it likely has dangerous chemicals. If it was made after 2013 most likely it is free of PCBs and PDBEs.
7. Drink clean water. Bottled water is not a great alternative because of the lack of testing on bottled water quality and the leaching that occurs from packaging materials. Choose a good water filter instead and invest in a few reusable water bottles.
8. When eating fish, choose wild-caught varieties, and grill or broil to burn off the fat that contains the most PCBs. Avoid larger fish, such as tuna, which have higher levels of mercury.

9. Eat an anti-inflammatory diet. In addition to the evidence showing that an anti-inflammatory diet reduces the risk of cardiovascular disease and metabolic syndrome, such a diet is likely to have a protective effect on overall health, including mitigating the damage from exposure to environmental chemicals.[4,5] Fruits and vegetables, especially cruciferous vegetables like broccoli, help to clear out toxins.
10. While the jury is still out regarding exposure to electromagnetic radiation and disease risk, use an earpiece when on your cellphone for prolonged periods of time, to decrease your brain's exposure to radiation I'd also avoid keeping your phone in your front pocket – if there is impact from EMF's at close range, why keep the device right next to your gonads?

Lastly, a word about mold. It is becoming clear that some people are more sensitive to negative effects from mold and the toxins they produce. Research suggests that certain genes cause some people to be more sensitive than others, so just because two people have the same amount of exposure, they may not be affected the same way. Symptoms of mold toxin exposure include frequent infections, brain fog, fatigue, and visual changes, among others. If you suspect that symptoms or illnesses you have are related to mold, there are testing kits that can be used to identify whether or not your home or office is contaminated.

The Bottom Line

Don't think it's all hype about health impacts from chemicals in our environment—the risks are real. Pesticides, chemicals in plastics, and flame retardants do impact our health, especially our hormonal health. So protect your sexual function and follow some of the tips listed in this chapter to decrease your exposure.

Notes

1. J. R. Rochester, "Bisphenol A and Human Health: A Review of the Literature," *Reproductive Toxicology* 42 (2013): 132–155, doi: 10.1016/j.reprotox.2013.08.008.
2. J. E. Lim et al., "Serum Persistent Organic Pollutants and Prostate Cancer Risk: A Case-Cohort Study," *International Journal of Hygiene and Environmental Health* 220, no. 5 (2017): 849–856, doi: 10.1016/j.ijheh.2017.03.014.

3. American Cancer Society, "Cellular Phones," https://www.cancer.org/cancer/cancer-causes/radiation-exposure/cellular-phones.html.
4. Frank B. Hu, "The Mediterranean Diet and Mortality—Olive Oil and Beyond," *New England Journal of Medicine* 348 (2003): 2595–2596, doi: 10.1056/NEJMp030069.
5. J. B. Hoffman and B. Hennig, "Protective Influence of Healthful Nutrition on Mechanisms of Environmental Pollutant Toxicity and Disease Risks," *Annals of the New York Academy of Sciences* 1398, no. 1 (2017): 99–107, doi: 10.1111/nyas.13365.

Resources

The following are great places to start learning more about how to avoid the risks of environmental toxins:

Home Environmental Health and Safety Assessment Tool, developed by A. Davis at the University of Maryland School of Nursing Environmental Health Education Center: https://envirn.org/wp-content/uploads/2017/03/davis-home-environmental-health-and-safety-assessment-tool.pdf.

Environmental Working Group's guide to pesticides and the "Dirty Dozen," those produce items most likely to have higher levels of pesticides: https://www.ewg.org/research/ewgs-dirty-dozen-cancer-prevention-edition#.WgTxYv9MGfA.

Environmental Working Group's guide to healthy cleaning: https://www.ewg.org/guides/cleaners#.WzlWV4plCfA

Environmental Working Group's guide to phthalate-free personal care products: https://www.ewg.org/skindeep.

The Natural Resources Defense Council frequently has tips on avoiding pesticides or chemical fertilizers, such as in the coffee you use: https://www.nrdc.org/stories/green-your-coffee-habit.

Pesticide Action Network, all the information you need about pesticides: panna.org.

The Monterey Bay Aquarium's guide to the safest seafood to eat: https://www.seafoodwatch.org/seafood-recommendations/consumer-guides.

Agency for Toxic Substances and Disease Registry, part of the Centers for Disease Control: www.ATSDR.cdc.gov.

SECTION 2

Specific Male Health Goals

Prevention and Integrative Approach to Treatment

8

Optimal Heart Health

You remember Pete. He's the guy who was at higher risk of having a heart attack not only because he was overweight and had high cholesterol but also because he had unfavorable genes. He underwent a CT scan that showed he had plaque in his coronary arteries, blocking blood flow to his heart muscle. When Pete learned just how high his risk was for a heart attack in the near future, that was a wake-up call for him, and he started taking care of his health.

While we often think of chest pain as a warning of heart problems, in fact more than half of sudden cardiac events (like heart attacks and strokes) occur in men with no prior symptoms.[1] And most occur in people with normal cholesterol, so having normal lab results isn't an indicator that you are out of the woods.

Heart disease is the number one killer of men. But when it comes to preventing heart disease, much of the power lies in our own hands (and our minds). Consider the INTERHEART study, published in 2004; this groundbreaking global study of 29,000 participants found that nine risk factors (listed in Box 8.1) account for over 90 percent of heart attack risk. In this study, men were more likely than women to have a heart attack before age sixty, but if you corrected for these nine risk factors, the gender difference nearly evaporated. Why is that so important? It shows that you can control your risk for a heart attack. Only 10 percent of the risk for a heart attack is

Box 8.1 These Nine Factors Account for Over 90 Percent of All Heart Attacks

1. Hypertension
2. Smoking
3. High cholesterol
4. Diabetes
5. Obesity
6. Poor diet
7. Low levels of physical activity
8. Too much alcohol
9. Stress or limited social support

genetic—it is mostly *not* built into your DNA as a male or as someone with a bad family history of heart disease. You can significantly minimize your risk of having a heart attack by modifying those nine factors listed in the box, even if you have "bad" genes.

In fact, according to a study from the University of Washington, two-thirds of the more than 600,000 annual deaths from cardiovascular disease in the United States could be prevented just by healthy eating. That's 400,000 deaths that could be prevented each year.[2] You could be one of those saved. It's not just about eating too much processed meat or refined sugar (although those are contributing factors). Many of these deaths were because of things guys *weren't* eating—namely, nuts and seeds, vegetables, whole grains, and fruit. It is entirely possible to significantly reduce your risk of dying from a heart attack by tweaking your eating habits.

Assessing Cardiovascular Risk

In order to be most effective at preventing cardiovascular disease, it is important to know who is at the highest risk. For someone at lower risk, we might be less strict about diet or the need to lose weight. But for someone who is at high risk, we will work hard to minimize all of the controllable risk factors as much as possible. Testing I recommend to improve our understanding of a patient's risk includes laboratory evaluation using advanced cardiac biomarkers as well as CT scanning to look for plaque (measured as a coronary calcium score) and carotid ultrasound. Let's look at some of these specific tests.

Advanced Testing for Heart Disease Risk

Advanced Cholesterol Panel

Historically, cholesterol measurement has been simplified into total cholesterol, LDL or "bad" cholesterol, HDL or "good" cholesterol, and triglycerides. Unfortunately, this does not tell the entire story of cholesterol-associated risk. An advanced cholesterol panel provides far more information.

LDL and HDL

Although high LDL and low HDL levels are certainly considered risk factors, most heart attacks occur in patients who have normal levels on the standard, less-precise tests for HDL and LDL. But not all LDL and HDL particles are created equal, and they don't all have the same degree of risk for causing plaque.

The vertical autoprofile (VAP) and other advanced heart disease risk panels, like NMR, offer a cholesterol profile measurement that simultaneously measures concentrations of all types of cholesterol, or lipoproteins. LDL actually consists of four density subclasses, LDL_1 through LDL_4, ranging from large, buoyant particles, which confer less risk, to small, dense particles, which are associated with higher risk. The difference in risk is because smaller, more dense particles are more easily oxidized (oxidative damage takes place as a result of daily living and overall inflammation) and thus taken up into the walls of the arteries around the heart, causing dangerous plaque buildup. Individuals vary in which size of LDL particle is more common in their blood, and knowing which type you are building up can help you to know how dangerous your cholesterol profile is. Buildup of even the worst type of LDL particles can be significantly modified through lifestyle changes as well as statins (medication that lowers cholesterol) or niacin therapy. HDL particles are also classified as more protective or less protective based upon size, starting at HDL_1, which is the most buoyant and the most protective, and ending with HDL_4, which is the densest and the least protective.

This lipoprotein subclass separation offers a direct measurement of LDL and HDL (rather than the typical calculated measure found in standard lipid panels), allowing us to better define risk and measure response to treatment.

CRP

C-reactive protein is a marker of inflammation. Plaque is much more likely to rupture and cause a stroke or heart attack if it is inflamed. Because of this, elevated CRP has been shown to increase the risk of heart attack, stroke, and sudden cardiac death. In fact, one very large study published in the *New England Journal of Medicine* showed that CRP was more effective at predicting heart attack risk than LDL cholesterol.[3] Exercise and weight loss, as well as statin use, have all been shown to decrease CRP levels. Individuals who have an elevated CRP despite normal lipids might still benefit from lowering cholesterol with dietary changes, medications, or supplements and would certainly benefit from an anti-inflammatory diet.

Lp(a)

Lipoprotein (a) is a cousin to cholesterol, similar in structure to LDL cholesterol. It is now considered to be a strong, independent, inheritable marker for coronary disease. Patients with an elevated Lp(a) level (despite having a normal LDL level) are considered at higher risk, so I would recommend more aggressive management of all the other risk factors mentioned here if your Lp(a) is high, adding supplements like niacin and antioxidant nutrients and considering a plant-based diet. You might recognize this marker from having heard about it when Bob Harper, the trainer from the TV show *The Biggest Loser*, had a heart attack. He had been in great shape and had normal cholesterol, but it turns out the culprit for him was high Lp(a).

ApoB

ApoB is considered an aggregate marker of all atherogenic (plaque-promoting) particles, including LDL, related particles called VLDL and IDL, and Lp(a). Higher levels of ApoB correlate with higher cardiovascular risk.

HgbA1c

We know that diabetes significantly increases cardiovascular disease risk, but it's not as if the increased risk starts only when someone is officially diagnosed with diabetes. The higher the blood sugar, the higher the risk. Hemoglobin A1c (HgbA1c) is the best assessment of blood sugar over time. It represents the average blood sugar over the three-month period before blood is drawn by measuring the percentage of red blood cells (which live around three months) with blood sugar molecules attached. Normal blood sugar would be reflected in a HgbA1C of around 5.0–5.4 percent. A value of 6.0 percent means you officially have prediabetes, and 6.5 percent confirms a diagnosis of diabetes. But anything above 5.5 percent increases the risk for developing diabetes and for diabetes-associated complications like heart disease.

ApoE Genetic Test

The ApoE gene codes for a protein called apolipoprotein E, which packages cholesterol and other fats to carry them through the blood stream. A certain form of this gene, ApoE4, causes the apolipoprotein to be less efficient, increasing your risk for atherosclerosis, and therefore for heart attack and stroke. (It also affects your risk for Alzheimer's disease; see Chapter 12.) This is the form of the gene that Pete has, as was mentioned in Chapter 2.

Homocysteine

This amino acid increases the risk for heart disease when it's elevated. This is part because high homocysteine is associated with low levels of vitamins B_6, B_{12}, and folate. High homocysteine contributes to increased inflammation and irritation of the blood vessels, increasing risk for atherosclerosis. Taking folate can lower homocysteine, but many people have an abnormal form of the MTHFR gene, making it important that they take a special form of folate, called methylated folate, in order to lower homocysteine to a safe range.

Advanced Imaging

Coronary Artery Calcium (CAC) Score

Traditionally, the exercise stress test has been used to predict risk of future heart attack. During a stress test, you generally exercise on a treadmill (or you may be given medication to make the heart work harder) in order to assess how the heart performs when stressed. If there are signs that the heart doesn't get enough blood flow when it's working harder, a condition called stress-induced ischemia, then further testing such as a coronary angiogram is performed to see where there might be blockage to blood flow. An angiogram is an invasive test that takes place in a specialized surgical-type suite; the cardiologist inserts a catheter into the groin and snakes it up into the blood vessels around the heart in order to inject dye that can reveal blockages. However, stress tests have their own limitations and often miss finding risky plaque, so the medical community is still debating which individuals will most benefit from stress testing.

Most cardiologists agree that one of the best and easiest tests to see if there is atherosclerosis (plaque buildup) in the arteries around the heart is the coronary calcium score. This test uses a CT scan to find calcium in coronary arteries, which is a good marker for actual plaque. Coronary calcium scores are classified into five groups: 0, no coronary calcium; 1–100, mild coronary calcium; 101–399, moderate calcification; 400–999, severe calcification; over 1,000, extensive calcification. The majority of coronary events, like heart attacks or sudden cardiac death (when the heart stops abruptly), occur in individuals who have a calcium score over 100. Studies have backed up the prognostic value of these scans.[4] It is important to acknowledge that not all atherosclerotic plaque is calcified and that the presence of a large amount of calcium does not prove the presence of significant stenoses (narrowing of arteries); that requires a coronary angiogram to confirm. In addition, there is a small although real risk from exposure to radiation during the CT scan, comparable to a screening mammogram.

CIMT/Duplex Ultrasound

Carotid intima-media thickness (CIMT) has long been used as a surrogate marker for cardiovascular disease and for the prevalence of atherosclerosis in other arteries in the body. It uses duplex ultrasound, which is noninvasive and painless. Elevated CIMT is associated with the development of heart disease and stroke. Currently, the American Heart Association recommends the use of CIMT screening in individuals who are at risk for cardiovascular disease. It is interesting to note that an increased CIMT is also correlated with erectile dysfunction, supporting the role of CIMT in assessing risk for atherosclerosis across the arterial system, including arteries to the brain and penis as well as the heart.

Lifestyle Change Intervention

In most of American health care today, the focus shifted long ago from treating every aspect of a patient's health to a disease-driven model. This means that treatment is focused on symptoms and disease, not the root causes of ill health or the prevention of diseases that have yet to develop. But making positive changes to one's lifestyle continues to be the single most effective way to prevent and treat most cardiovascular diseases. It's not just about lowering cholesterol with diet and medications. All cardiovascular disease is closely related not only to cholesterol but also to overall inflammation, which causes any cholesterol plaque that exists to be more likely to cause problems. Inflammation is a direct result of obesity, poor nutrition, exposure to toxins, a sedentary lifestyle, and high levels of stress.

An integrative approach to heart health broadens the traditional diagnosis and treatment of disease utilizing both Western-style diagnostic tests and medications when needed along with a broader focus on all aspects of health, including nutrition, exercise, and psychosocial stress. One program that incorporates all of these elements plus a focus on social/community support is the Ornish Program for Reversing Heart Disease. Developed by Dr. Dean Ornish of the prestigious University of California, San Francisco Medical Center, it is the first program scientifically proven to reverse heart disease by optimizing these four areas. The program includes eighteen 4-hour sessions, incorporating information about a whole-foods plant-based diet, stress management training, physical exercise, and group emotional support. It has been so successful at reversing heart disease among people with ongoing angina (chest pain from blocked coronary arteries) that it has been proven to be as good as surgical interventions such as placing a stent or bypass surgery. It is covered by Medicare and some insurance companies.[5]

Nutrition

What you put into your mouth can directly affect your cardiovascular health. One of the first steps to take is to look at overall weight, as obesity is extremely common in the United States, and being overweight has been proven over and over again to increase the chance of having a heart attack. Beyond simply maintaining a healthy weight, limiting saturated fats from animal foods (the fat in dairy, red meat, and animal skin) can lower dangerous LDL cholesterol. However, when you simply replace saturated animal fats with carbohydrates, there is only a very small reduction in cardiovascular risk. In contrast, replacing saturated fats (such as in red meat) with monounsaturated or polyunsaturated fats (from foods like nuts, fish, olives, and avocados) was associated with an almost tenfold greater decrease in risk.[6]

There are two types of diets that have been especially proven to lower heart disease risk. One is the Mediterranean diet, which is high in monounsaturated fats. Foods rich in this type of healthy fat include olive oil, canola oil, many types of nuts, and avocados. (See Table 8.1.) The Mediterranean diet also includes large amounts of fresh fruits and vegetables; wholegrain rather than refined carbohydrates; low to moderate amounts of dairy, fish, and poultry; low amounts of red meat; minimal amounts of processed foods; and a low to moderate amount of wine.

The other type of diet that has been proven to lower risk is a low-fat whole-foods plant-based diet, such as the one used in the Ornish Reversal program. While such a diet is a powerful way to maximize the chance of

Table 8.1: Fats That Decrease Heart Disease Risk, and Fats That Increase It

Effect on Heart Disease Risk	Type of Fat	Food Sources
Decrease risk	Monounsaturated fats	Olive oil, canola oil, nuts (macadamias, hazlenuts and pecans), avocados
	Polyunsaturated fats	Fish, flaxseed oil, walnuts, almonds
Increase risk	Saturated animal fats	Dairy fat, egg yolk, poultry skin, red meat
May decrease risk, but evidence still unclear	Saturated plant fats	Coconut oil

preventing heart disease and many cancers, a diet that emphasizes plant-based foods need not be an all-or-nothing option, as limiting intake of animal protein and fat to any extent while increasing intake of plant-based foods will be beneficial.

The last thing I'll say about fats is that the polyunsaturated omega-3 fats, most prevalent in fish but also found in walnuts and almonds, have been shown to be strongly correlated with a decrease in LDL cholesterol, inflammation, and heart disease risk. Hence, eating fish (while watching out for species with high mercury content) or taking a supplement of omega-3s is recommended for most people at any risk of heart disease. Doses of 1,000–2,000 mg of the combination of the two active types of omega 3 fatty acids, EPA (eicosapentaenoic acid) and DHA (docosahexaenoic acid), have been shown to reduce risk of heart attack or recurrence of heart attack and to help in heart failure.[7]

What about carbs, especially sugar? There are conflicting reports as to which is worse, saturated fat or sugar, in terms of increasing inflammation and worsening risk for heart disease. The bottom line: limit both if you want to be healthy. Natural sugars, found in fruits, vegetables, and whole grains, are not to be feared. But processed sugar and sweeteners, especially high-fructose corn syrup and other syrups made from agave, rice, or corn, contribute to high blood sugar levels, which promote fat storage, insulin resistance and inflammation. There is compelling evidence that sugar is actually more of a risk for heart disease than fat, because sugar causes the liver to build up a type of fat that is worse for the heart than dietary fat.[8] This is not to say that "butter is back," as we saw a few years ago on the covers of some national popular magazines; animal-based saturated fat is still not healthy, but neither is added sugar.

Finally, there's dietary fiber. High-fiber diets have been shown to minimize constipation, increase satiety, slow glucose absorption from the small intestine, and inhibit cholesterol absorption from the small intestine, thereby reducing blood cholesterol levels. Furthermore, two of the largest and most respected studies of the effect of diet on health, the Nurses' Health Study and the Health Professionals' Follow-up Study, showed reduced risk of both fatal and nonfatal heart attack in both men and women who had the highest fiber intake compared to those who had the lowest.[9,10] For example, eating beans, which are generally high in fiber, four times a week has been shown to lower the risk of heart disease by more than 20 percent.

ON BEANS

Are beans good for you or bad for you? It is very confusing that some popular diets, such as Whole 30 and paleo, eschew beans for the most part. I, and most nutrition experts, disagree with leaving them out of your diet. Beans are filling, healthy sources of protein and fiber and are common components of the healthiest diets in the world, such as those in areas known as the Blue Zones, where people are healthier than anywhere else on earth. Whole 30 and paleo proponents argue that beans contain phytates, substances that can block absorption of certain essential nutrients. But in order to get high enough levels of phytates to cause a problem, you'd have to eat raw beans in large amounts, as soaking and cooking reduce phytates by a lot. Furthermore, many, many foods, including foods allowed by these diets, have as much or more phytates than beans. Until there is some new, surprising evidence that cooked beans in the amounts generally eaten cause any health problem, I'd continue eating them.

Exercise

A sedentary life is detrimental to good health. Period. Almost all cardiovascular diseases and diabetes have been shown to worsen in patients with sedentary lives. The Health Professionals' Follow-up Study evaluated 44,452 men and demonstrated that the risk for death decreased as the amount of physical activity increased.

A provocative study looking at exercise versus stent placement in patients with coronary artery disease showed that daily exercise over a twelve-month period offered just as much improvement in symptoms of angina (chest pain) as stents. This is why exercise is included in the Ornish Reversal plan and why most patients who have had a cardiac event are referred to a cardiac rehab exercise program. Why not start the program *before* the event, instead of waiting for it to happen, with potentially disastrous consequences?

Box 8.2 5 Minutes to Exercise

This exercise program is meant for people who are "exercise
resistant." The goal is to first focus on creating an exercise
routine, then work on increasing the effort. This program
is meant to be very simple and basic and therefore easy to
accomplish.

- Exercise for only 5 minutes—but do it *every* day (don't skip
  any days).
- Don't exercise for more than 5 minutes.
- Exercise at any pace.
- If you get bored, then increase the pace—not the time. Keep it at
  5 minutes.
- If you're sick or tired, slow down the pace—but don't skip the
  exercise.
- After the first month, increase the duration by 5 minutes, so that
  you're exercising for 10 minutes—every day.
- Increase the duration by 5 minutes each month after that.
  - When you get to 30 minutes, you can drop down to 4 days a
    week, but increase each month by 5 minutes until you get to
    40 minutes a day for four days a week.

Ideally, aerobic exercise should be combined with muscle-building activity at least three times per week for at least 40 minutes per session.[11]
However, even mild to moderate levels of exercise have a significant impact
on cardiovascular mortality. Box 8.2 lists an easy way to slowly build up to a
heart-healthy exercise routine.

Supplements

A number of vitamins and supplements have been shown to be of benefit in
preventing cardiovascular disease (see Table 8.2). It is important that you
discuss any supplements with your physician, who can help you tailor what
you take to your particular risks and to make sure none of them interact
with medications you may be taking.

Table 8.2

Supplement	How It Helps in Heart Disease	Dose	Comments
Omega-3 fatty acids (from fish oil)	Decreases mortality, prevents arrhythmias, lowers triglycerides	2,000 mg EPA + DHA (combined) daily	Decreases inflammation.
Coenzyme Q10	Helps to treat congestive heart failure and statin-induced myopathy (muscle pain from statins or red yeast rice)	50–200 mg daily	Statins deplete CoQ10 levels.
Magnesium	Decreases arrhythmias and helps control hypertension	250–1,000 mg daily, depending on formulation (chelated and Slow-Mag are best absorbed)	Dose-dependent lowering of blood pressure. Best taken at night because it may cause drowsiness; also can cause loose stools.
Hawthorn	Helps to treat congestive heart failure	900–1,800 mg of standardized extract daily	May improve heart function and exercise tolerance. May reduce symptoms associated with heart failure.

Psychological Risk Factors in the Development of Cardiovascular Disease

You may be tempted to skip over this section, but evidence of the connection between the mind and body is some of the most exciting news that has come along since I graduated from medical school. Remember the INTERHEART study, mentioned at the beginning of this chapter, showing that nine risk factors were found to account for 90 percent of the risk for heart disease in men? Of these risk factors, psychosocial factors, including depression, stress, and anxiety, were found to increase the risk of heart disease more than most other traditional risk factors, including hypertension, diabetes, and obesity.[12]

Although stress may at times be an adaptive response to ensure survival, stress hormones—most notably epinephrine, cortisol, and aldosterone—are associated with impaired glucose metabolism, weight gain, arrhythmia, hypertension, hyperlipidemia, inflammation, and coronary spasm. In addition, stress can adversely affect blood vessel tone, immune function, coagulation, and the perception of pain. Individuals who experience high mental stress in their daily life have twice the risk of myocardial ischemia (reduced blood flow to the heart) than people with less stress. And experiencing high levels of anger over an extended period of time was found to increase the risk of heart attack by 230 percent!

A growing body of evidence also suggests that depression may predispose people to cardiovascular events. Depression is common after a heart attack and is associated with an increased risk of mortality for at least eighteen months afterward.[13] This aspect of mental health is often underdiagnosed and inadequately treated, but notice that stress management and social support are both important aspects of the Ornish Reversal plan, which has been so well proven to reverse heart disease.

Evidence-Based Mind-Body Therapies

What sort of stress management has been proven to make a difference in terms of heart disease risk? A study published in the *Journal of the American Medical Association* demonstrated that biofeedback and progressive muscle relaxation cut in half the risk of having a cardiovascular event over a five-year period.[14] Biofeedback uses monitoring of physiological markers such as heart rate, blood pressure, skin temperature, and muscle tension to train people to change habitual reactions to stress. It usually

Table 8.2 continued

Supplement	How It Helps in Heart Disease	Dose	Comments
β-sitosterol (sterol/ stanol), aka plant sterols	Lowers cholesterol	800–2,000 mg daily	
Soluble fiber	Lowers cholesterol and helps with weight loss	1.5 g daily	
Red yeast rice	Lowers cholesterol in a similar way to statins	1,200 mg twice daily	Significant product variability— many red yeast rice products don't contain the amount of active ingredient (monacolin) needed to lower cholesterol. Check brand quality or take a statin instead.
Vitamin D	Low levels are associated with increased heart disease risk	Amount depends on blood levels of 25-hydroxy vitamin D_3	Use vitamin D_3 (cholecalciferol) rather than D_2 (ergocalciferol) for better absorption.

displays visual or auditory feedback to raise patients' awareness of their bodily responses and to train them to consciously control those responses using various relaxation techniques such as deep breathing and muscle relaxation. Progressive muscle relaxation involves focusing on each body part in turn, tightening and then relaxing each muscle group, working up the body from toes to head. There are dozens of YouTube videos that can talk you through guided progressive muscle relaxation.

Mindfulness meditation, which focuses on moment-to-moment awareness, usually through concentrating on the breath, has been shown to reduce stress scores and help with sleep and mood. There are many ways to learn mindfulness techniques, from in-person mindfulness-based stress reduction (MBSR) training based on the seminal work of Jon Kabat-Zinn to apps like Calm and Headspace (see Chapter 6 for information on all these). Another form of meditation, called Transcendental Meditation (TM), became popular in the late 1960s. It involves mantra-based meditation for 20 minutes twice a day, and studies have demonstrated improvement in hypertension and cardiovascular morbidity and mortality in patients who practice TM daily. Furthermore, TM has been shown to improve not only blood pressure but also insulin resistance.[15]

Powerful Mind-Body Tools to Prevent Heart Disease

Mindfulness-based stress reduction (MBSR)

Transcendental Meditation

Biofeedback

Progressive muscle relaxation

Journaling on gratitude

Let's go back to my patient, Pete, with whom we started this chapter. Peter had a wake-up call when a CT scan showed significant amounts of plaque in his arteries. He realized that he needed to make some meaningful changes in order to prevent "the big one." He agreed to enroll in the Ornish Reversal program, which had him work on his stress with meditation, start an exercise program, and, with the support of nutritionists, change his diet to a lower-fat, more plant-based one. He also benefited from the group discussions about how hard it is to change all of these behaviors. He, like the other participants, found it helpful to make these changes along with others in the same boat and with the help of coaches. He managed to lose twenty pounds in the eighteen weeks of the program. His blood pressure and blood sugar both came down to normal ranges. The only medication he still needed to take was a statin to keep his cholesterol down. The best part was that Pete truly felt better. He had more energy to play basketball with his son and was less easily agitated in general. He is sticking to the diet and continuing to do some daily meditation using an app on his smartphone.

An Integrative Approach to Cardiovascular Disease

A checkup with a practitioner like myself who takes an integrative approach to cardiac health will look different from the traditional standard American physical in several ways. First, in addition to taking the usual vital signs (pulse rate, temperature, blood pressure), the practitioner will measure your waist circumference and calculate your body mass index. These will be recorded so that your progress can be tracked over time.

The provider will ask about what really matters to you. This may seem silly, but homing in on what matters to you—your sense of purpose—reveals what motivates you. Beyond just not wanting to die, what do you want to be working toward? In what exact ways would having heart problems affect your life? It is important to be very clear about how your health affects your ability to accomplish your goals. I may recommend some fairly big changes in your lifestyle: changing your diet substantially, starting an exercise program, and maybe starting a meditation practice. This all requires quite a bit of motivation, so it's important that you are clear on what you want your health *for*. That's what will keep you motivated.

A thorough history of your health and an accurate family history are then taken. The practitioner will not only ask about chest pain or shortness of breath but also ask specific questions about daily exercise, diet, alcohol consumption, and life stressors and coping skills. This is followed by a physical exam.

Next we have the labs. I recommend obtaining an advanced cholesterol panel (NMR, VAP, or similar), CRP, HgbA1c, Lp(a), ApoB, homocysteine, vitamin D level, comprehensive metabolic panel, and complete blood count. Ideally I would include genetic tests such as ApoE to determine whether or not you have genes that can significantly increase your heart disease risk. Because we are focusing on heart health, I would want to do a CT scan to determine your coronary calcium score.

After a review of your test results along with your health and family history, your own personalized risk can be determined and a customized plan can be created for you. If you are like most American men over fifty, you are at relatively high risk for heart disease. Your plan might look like this:

Diet: whole-foods plant-based Mediterranean-style diet.
Supplements:
Omega-3 fatty acids as fish oil, 2,000 mg a day of EPA + DHA combined
Vitamin D_3 (if testing reveals a low level)
Coenzyme Q10, 100 mg a day
Magnesium gluconate, 400 mg at night
Methylfolate, 400 mcg a day (if you have unfavorable MTHFR genes)
Exercise: Starting slow, with 5 minutes a day, and increasing the duration of each exercise period by 5 minutes each month until you're exercising for 40 minutes a day at least 4 days a week
Stress management: A mindfulness program like MBSR or daily use of a meditation app.

The Bottom Line

Many of my patients fear having a heart attack, because they know it's the number one killer of men. But you have more control over this happening than you think. Be proactive by having your risk assessed in the ways described in this chapter and implementing the changes discussed here.

Questions to Ask Your Doctor

1. What's my risk for having a heart attack in the next five years? (Your doctor can answer that, but not without data. I recommend asking your doctor about the advanced tests discussed in this chapter. Insurance may not cover all of them, so ask what your out-of-pocket costs would be. If you have the tests, your doctor should be able to interpret the results to guide you on your next steps.)
2. What supplements can I try that might help lower my risk? (Before starting on medications for something like high cholesterol, talk to your doctor about a trial of intensive lifestyle change and supplements for a few months.)

Notes

1. D. Lloyd-Jones et al., "Heart Disease and Stroke Statistics—2010 Update. A Report from the American Heart Association Statistics Committee and Stroke Statistics Subcommittee," *Circulation* 121 (2010): e1–e170, doi: 10.1161/circulationaha.109.192667.
2. American Heart Association, "Unhealthy Diets Linked to More than 400,000 Cardiovascular Deaths," ScienceDaily, March 9, 2017, www.sciencedaily.com/releases/2017/03/170309142345.htm.
3. P. M. Ridker et al., "Comparison of CRP and LDL in the Prediction of First Cardiovascular Events," *New England Journal of Medicine* 347 (2002): 1557–1565, doi: 10.1056/NEJMoa021993.
4. Multi-Ethnic Study of Atherosclerosis website, www.mesa-nhlbi.org.
5. "Undo It with Ornish: Ornish Lifestyle Medicine," https://www.ornish.com/undo-it.
6. F. B. Hu et al., "Dietary Fat Intake and the Risk of Coronary Heart Disease in Women," *New England Journal of Medicine* 337 (1997): 1491.
7. David S. Siscovick et al., "Omega-3 Polyunsaturated Fatty Acid (Fish Oil) Supplementation and the Prevention of Clinical Cardiovascular Disease," *Circulation* 135 (2017): e867–e884, doi: 10.1161/CIR.0000000000000482.
8. Q. Yang et al., "Added Sugar Intake and Cardiovascular Diseases Mortality Among US Adults," *JAMA Internal Medicine* 174, no. 4 (2014): 516–524, doi: 10.1001/jamainternmed.2013.13563.
9. E. B. Rimm et al., "Vegetable, Fruit, and Cereal Fiber Intake and Risk of Coronary Heart Disease Among Men," *Journal of the American Medical Association* 275, no. 6 (1996): 447–451.
10. A. Wolk et al., "Long-Term Intake of Dietary Fiber and Decreased Risk of Coronary Heart Disease Among Women," *Journal of the American Medical Association* 281, no. 21 (1999): 1998–2004.
11. P. D. Thompson et al., "Exercise and Physical Activity in the Prevention and Treatment of Atherosclerotic Cardiovascular Disease: A Statement from the Council on Clinical Cardiology," *Circulation* 107 (2003): 3109–3116.
12. S. Yusuf, S. Hawken, and S. Ounpuu, "Effect of Potentially Modifiable Risk Factors Associated with Myocardial Infarction in 52 Countries (the INTERHEART Study): Case-Control Study," *Lancet* 364 (2004): 937–952.
13. N. Frasure-Smith, F. Lesperance, and M. Talajic, "Depression and 18-Month Prognosis After Myocardial Infarction," *Circulation* 91 (1995): 999–1005.

14. J. A. Blumenthal et al., "Effects of Exercise and Stress Management Training on Markers of Cardiovascular Risk in Patients with Ischemic Heart Disease: A Randomized Controlled Trial," *Journal of the American Medical Association* 293 (2005): 1626–1634.
15. R. H. Schneider et al., "Long-Term Effects of Stress Reduction on Mortality in Persons > 55 Years of Age with Systemic Hypertension," *American Journal of Cardiology* 95 (2005): 1060–1064.

Resources

Apps for mindfulness training:

> Calm
> Headspace
> 10% Happier
> Insight Timer

Books:

> *Full Catastrophe Living: How to Cope with Stress, Pain, and Illness Using Mindfulness Meditation*, by Jon Kabat-Zinn
> *How Not to Die: Discover the Foods Scientifically Proven to Prevent and Reverse Disease*, by Michael Gregor with Gene Stone
> *Healthy Aging: A Lifelong Guide to Your Well-Being*, by Andrew Weil
> *Undo It! How Simple Lifestyle Change Can Reverse Most Chronic Disease*, by Dean Ornish and Anne Ornish

Websites:

> The latest science on diet: NutritionFacts.org
> Ornish Lifestyle Medicine: Ornish.com
> Dr. Spar's website on optimal health for men: DrSpar.com

9

The Prostate and Optimal Health

Jason: Enlarged Prostate

Jason is a fifty-eight-year-old healthy man who has been having trouble sleeping. He falls asleep well, but lately he has been having to get up three or four times during the night to urinate. Then it takes him a bit to fall back asleep. In addition, during the day he gets very strong urges to urinate and feels he has to get to a bathroom quickly or he might lose bladder control. He goes to his doctor to see what he can do. His doctor performs a digital rectal exam and remarks that Jason's prostate is over twice as large as normal.

Of course Jason's biggest fear is that he could have prostate cancer. But it is actually more likely that he has a noncancerous enlargement of the gland called benign prostatic hypertrophy (BPH).

Prostate issues are one of the most common concerns among my patients. BPH, which affects half of men over the age of sixty, causes urinary issues such as urgency, less forceful stream, or waking up multiple times at night to urinate. This chapter will focus primarily on noncancerous conditions of the prostate, including BPH and chronic prostatitis/chronic pelvic pain syndrome (CP/CPPS). Prostate cancer will be discussed in Chapter 10, on cancer in general, since integrative medicine prevention approaches for prostate cancer are much the same as the approaches used to prevent cancer elsewhere in the body.

For BPH, after cancer is ruled out, there are multiple approaches for treatment. Several categories of medication can be used to treat BPH: alpha blockers, 5-alpha-reductase inhibitors, and PDE5-inhibitors. Table 9.1 lists these medications. Alpha blockers prevent the nervous system from overstimulating the prostate, and 5-alpha-reductase inhibitors block the conversion of testosterone into dihydrotestosterone (DHT), the form of the hormone that contributes to BPH. PDE5-inhibitors are the class of medications used for erectile dysfunction (ED), including the drugs Viagra (sildenafil) and Cialis (tadalafil). Cialis has been shown to be effective for BPH when taken daily at a dose less than that used for ED (5 mg vs. 20 mg). These medications can be very helpful and have been shown to reduce the need for surgery, but they do have side effects that can limit their tolerability.

Botanical Alternatives

There are botanicals (Table 9.2) that can effectively treat BPH, with some working the same way as pharmaceuticals do, often with fewer side effects. Saw palmetto is probably the most-studied botanical for BPH. It inhibits the conversion of testosterone into DHT in a similar way as the 5-alpha reductase inhibitors. It also slows growth of prostate tissue. The main active constituent is a compound called beta-sitosterol, which can be used on its own. Saw palmetto has been shown to be as effective as Proscar (finasteride) and efficacious enough to reduce the need for BPH surgery.[1] Another botanical, pygeum, has a similar mechanism of action; however, pygeum comes from the bark of an African tree and is overharvested, so unless you can be sure it comes from a sustainable source, I do not recommend

Table 9.1 Medications for BPH

Category	Generic Name	Brand Name	Side Effects
Alpha blocker	Doxazosin	Cardura	Dizziness, light-headedness
Alpha blocker	Terazosin	Hytrin	Dizziness, light-headedness
Alpha blocker	Tamsulosin	Flomax	Ejaculatory effects; eye-related problems (floppy iris syndrome)
Alpha blocker	Alfuzosin	Uroxatral	Dizziness, light-headedness
Alpha blocker	Silodosin	Rapaflo	Some light-headedness
5-alpha-reductase inhibitor	Finasteride	Proscar	Erectile dysfunction, ejaculatory effects
5-alpha-reductase inhibitor	Dutasteride	Avodart	Erectile dysfunction, ejaculatory effects
PDE5 inhibitor	Tadalafil	Cialis	Light-headedness, tachycardia, low blood pressure

Table 9.2 Table of Botanicals

Botanical	Dose	Possible Interactions or side effects
Saw palmetto	320 mg daily (ideally 160 mg twice daily); allow 8 weeks before symptoms may improve	Increases blood-thinning effect of Plavix (clopidogrel) and Coumadin (warfarin); possible gastrointestinal symptoms
Nettle root	360 mg daily	Can cause blood thinning and reduce efficacy of some diabetes medications, so ask your doctor if taking medications for diabetes
Beta-sitosterol	60–65 mg 2 or 3 times daily	Gastrointestinal upset
Pumpkin seed	320 mg daily	Lower blood pressure
Lycopene	20–30 mg daily	
Rye pollen extract	126 mg 3 times daily	Gastrointestinal upset

using it, as there is no real advantage over saw palmetto and it threatens survival of the tree species. Combination formulas may include more than one botanical, such as saw palmetto with nettle root, which can be especially effective, as nettle root inhibits aromatase, the enzyme that converts testosterone to estrogen.

In addition to botanicals, zinc at a dose of 30 mg a day can help with BPH symptoms, especially for men on ACE inhibitors for blood pressure, a class of medications that can lower serum zinc levels. Caffeine and products that act as stimulants (including decongestants) may worsen BPH symptoms.

Stress and the Prostate

Several studies show a correlation between prostate health and stress. Higher levels of prostate-specific antigen (PSA) were found in those with greater stress, and in men with BPH, both prostate size and residual urine in the bladder after urinating (post-void volume) were associated with prolonged, lifelong stress. Higher stress causes activation of the sympathetic nervous system and its resultant hormones, epinephrine and norepinephrine, which have been implicated both in the increase in the size of the prostate and in the worsening of symptoms by leading to increased contraction of the pelvic floor and the prostate, thus stimulating the need to urinate.

Reducing chronic stress, therefore, is an important component in prevention and treatment of BPH. This may involve any of the techniques discussed elsewhere in this book (and especially in Chapter 6), including mindfulness meditation and breath work.

Exercise and the Prostate

Men who are more physically active are less likely to suffer from BPH, plain and simple. Even moderate activity, like walking regularly, can help. This is based on questionnaires completed by more than 30,000 men in the Health Professionals Follow-up Study, one of the largest and most respected studies on men's health.[2] By the way, those who exercised more also had less likelihood of erectile dysfunction.

Diet and the Prostate

The same recommendations for a healthful diet made elsewhere in this book, especially the benefits of a Mediterranean-style anti-inflammatory diet, apply to prostate health. Eating more fruits and vegetables, minimizing refined grains and added sugars, limiting meat consumption, choosing healthier fats, and avoiding hydrogenated fats (trans fats) help improve prostate health. The number one dietary approach to lessening the risk for BPH and also for prostate cancer is to maintain a healthy weight. Being overweight is one of the strongest risk factors for both of these conditions.

Complementary Medicine Approaches

Whole-systems approaches such as Ayurvedic medicine and traditional Chinese medicine (TCM) can also be helpful and are discussed in Chapters 15 and 16. While we can't identify the exact cause of BPH using typical Western medical understanding, these traditions treat underlying imbalances in the whole body, rather than just focusing on relieving symptoms. With both of these whole-systems approaches, treatment might include herbs, movement, and dietary recommendations. TCM might also include acupuncture or tai chi, both powerful modalities that can improve symptoms of BPH.

Preventing BPH

How can one prevent BPH from happening in the first place? We know that obesity and elevated blood sugar increase the risk of BPH through a cascade of events that results in prostate cell growth. Of course, high blood sugar is inflammatory, increasing a process that contributes to BPH symptoms. So maintaining a healthy weight and blood sugar helps prevent BPH. Studies have shown that light to moderate alcohol consumption can decrease the risk of BPH, while having more than seven alcoholic drinks per week increases risk.[3] Treating elevated cholesterol can also help BPH symptoms, especially through the use of omega-3 fatty acids or beta-sitosterol (the latter treats BPH both directly as well as through its cholesterol-lowering effects). Foods rich in the natural sterols that help BPH include green leafy vegetables, rice bran, wheat germ, peanuts, almonds and other nuts, and soybeans. Lastly, avoiding environmental exposures from pesticides and certain substances in plastics, which have hormonal effects, can help prevent BPH.

MINIMIZING BPH

The majority of men will develop prostate issues, such as BPH, as they age. But you can be proactive in order to prevent problems.

- Maintain a healthy diet (an anti-inflammatory diet)—this is one of the most effective ways to avoid prostate problems. Especially include these foods:
  - Fish rich in omega-3 fatty acids, like wild salmon
  - Tomatoes, rich in lycopene, which is best absorbed when the tomatoes are cooked and mixed with healthy oils, such as olive oil
  - Berries, rich in antioxidants
  - Broccoli, rich in antioxidants
  - Nuts, rich in zinc
  - Onions and garlic, with high allium content

Try to limit these:
  - Red meat (and when you do eat it, choose grass-fed meat and eat it at most twice a week)
  - Dairy, associated with increased risk of BPH
  - Caffeine, no more than 1–2 cups of caffeinated drinks a day
  - Alcohol, no more than 1–2 drinks a day and not more than 7 a week
  - Sodium, minimizing how much salt you add to foods and avoiding processed foods
- Maintain a healthy weight. Obesity is perhaps the strongest risk factor for all common prostate problems.
- Stay physically active. Cardiovascular exercise reduces risk for prostate problems.

Chronic Prostatitis/Chronic Pelvic Pain Syndrome (CP/CPPS)

ED: CHRONIC PROSTATITIS

Ed is a thirty-year-old active man who has had an aching pain in his pelvic area for a few months. It seems to be worse when he urinates, but his urine shows no sign of any infection, including STDs such as gonorrhea and chlamydia. He feels a little unwell overall and has had some issues with erectile dysfunction and decreased libido, which is unusual for him. His doctor examines his prostate; it's normal in size but a little tender. They try thirty days of antibiotics, but Ed's symptoms don't improve. Ed hasn't sustained any injuries that could explain the pelvic pain. A urologist diagnoses Ed with chronic prostatitis.

Chronic prostatitis affects an estimated 9 percent of men in the United States. Usually it is not caused by an infection, and in that way it is akin to the condition of chronic pelvic pain found in women, so the condition has come to be known more accurately as chronic prostatitis/chronic pelvic pain syndrome. Symptoms usually include intermittent pain in the pelvic or rectal area or even the urethra, which may be accompanied by generalized fatigue, depression, and urinary symptoms similar to BPH symptoms. Sexual issues, such as erectile dysfunction and problems with ejaculation, are also frequently experienced by men suffering from this condition. Unfortunately, there is no clear cause or simple recommendation for treatment.

Symptoms of CPPS

- Pain anywhere in the pelvis, including urethral pain (pain in the penis or at the tip), rectal pain, pain between the anus and rectum (the perineum), or testicular pain
- Urinary urgency
- Urinary frequency
- Burning sensation with urination
- Erectile dysfunction
- Abnormal ejaculation or pain after ejaculation

The first course of action when experiencing any of these symptoms is to be evaluated by a primary care practitioner or urologist. The doctor will first make sure there is no infection that would need to be treated with antibiotics. If there is an infection in the prostate, it is often treated with an extended course of antibiotics—because there is a protective barrier around the prostate that is meant to protect semen from toxins, it can take a while for sufficient concentrations of antibiotics to permeate the whole gland .

But in 90 percent of cases, no infection or even evidence of inflammation is found—we simply can't identify the cause. We do know, however, that smoking, higher alcohol consumption, and being overweight are associated with CP/CPPS, though we're not sure about the exact mechanism that links them.

Treatments

Some medications have been shown to be helpful, including alpha blockers (such as those in Table 9.1), anti-inflammatories (such as ibuprofen and naproxen), and some muscle relaxants. Plant-based therapies such as rye pollen extract and quercetin have also been shown to be helpful. Pollen therapy helps reduce muscle tightness and inflammation, especially in

The Prostate

prostate tissue. Quercetin is a powerful antioxidant that, especially when combined with the enzymes bromelain and papain, resulted in dramatic improvement in symptoms.[4] Lastly, I will mention that medical cannabis was helpful in over half of men in a Canadian study, who reported improvements in mood, painful muscle spasms, fatigue, and urinary symptoms.[5]

A review of studies of therapies for CP/CPPS found that certain dietary changes, such as consuming less spicy foods and caffeine and taking in more water and fiber, helped symptoms.[6] Exercise has also been shown to be helpful.

Some of the most helpful treatments include interventions such as myofascial physical therapy, acupuncture, and stress-management-focused cognitive behavioral therapy. This is because most men with CP/CPPS also suffer from some element of depression, anxiety, or panic disorder, all of which are worsened by stress and all of which worsen pain syndromes in general. Thus it is essential to use an integrated approach for successful treatment of this condition.

Chinese medicine, and particularly acupuncture, has been shown to be more effective than anti-inflammatory drugs or antibiotics for CP/CPPS. Interestingly, its impact is durable, meaning the effectiveness lasts beyond the end of the acupuncture treatments themselves.

The type of physical therapy that works for CPPS can be intense, because it involves the practitioner manually compressing trigger points in the area around the rectum, prostate, and genitals. If you can find an experienced professional trained in pelvic rehabilitation, it can be immensely helpful, even if it is painful during treatment. You just need to find a therapist trained specifically in this condition and in treating this sensitive part of the body.

Prostate Cancer

This chapter purposely focuses on noncancerous conditions of the prostate. I cover general cancer prevention in Chapter 10 and will touch on some specific issues regarding prostate cancer there. But I know there is a high level of concern among men about the possibility of being diagnosed with this disease. This is understandable, since prostate cancer is the most common cancer in men. Unfortunately, the screening tools that are available aren't great. The main screening blood test, for PSA, is controversial. Even the American Cancer Society and the U.S. Preventive Services Task

Force say that PSA screening should be considered and discussed with men but not necessarily done because it is overly sensitive.[7]

What is important to keep in mind regarding prostate cancer is this:

- While one in seven men will be diagnosed with prostate cancer, the vast majority of the time it is localized and slow-growing, allowing the patient and doctor an opportunity to consider treatment options or even consider simply monitoring closely for a period of time before undertaking treatment.
- Your family history, age (older men have more risk), race (people with African ancestry are at higher risk), and genes affect your chances of having prostate cancer. It's worth discussing your specific risk with your doctor. Consider genetic testing if you have many family members with hormonally related cancers such as prostate, ovarian, or breast cancer, as these can be related to the BRCA1 and BRCA2 genes.
- Maintaining a healthy weight is one of the most effective ways to minimize your risk.

The Bottom Line

Benign prostate conditions such as BPH and CP/CPPS are common and are especially well suited to treatment with integrative medicine approaches. In the case of BPH, many supplements are as beneficial as prescription medications, with fewer side effects, and offer the possibility of avoiding the need for surgical treatment. With CP/CPPS, there are simply no adequate Western medical treatments, but a combination approach of natural supplements, mind-body practice, and manual therapy intervention can lead to dramatic reduction in pain and improvement in quality of life.

Questions to Ask Your Doctor

1. Is it normal to wake up two or three times a night to urinate? (No, it's not. If you are waking up more than once at night to urinate, bring this up. You should have your prostate examined to see if it is enlarged.)
2. Should I be screened for prostate cancer? (If you are over fifty years old, or over forty with a close relative who was diagnosed with prostate cancer, or if you have African ancestry, ask about screening for prostate

cancer. At a minimum, you should have your prostate examined. You can discuss PSA and genetic testing as well.)

3. What can I do about the feeling that if I don't get to the bathroom quickly enough, I'll urinate on myself? (If you are having symptoms of BPH, such as urgency, change in urine flow, or urinating a lot, bring it up. Ask about the supplements mentioned in this chapter and consider trying them for a few months before starting medications.)

Notes

1. F. Hizli and M. C. Uygur, "A Prospective Study of the Efficacy of *Serenoa repens*, Tamsulosin, and *Serenoa repens* Plus Tamsulosin Treatment for Patients with Benign Prostate Hyperplasia," *International Urology and Nephrology* 39 (2007): 879–886, doi: 10.1007/s11255-006-9106-5.

2. E. A. Platz et al., "Physical Activity and Benign Prostatic Hyperplasia," *Archives of Internal Medicine* 158 (1998): 2349–2356.

3. A. Sierksma et al., "Effect of Moderate Alcohol Consumption on Plasma Dehydroepiandrosterone Sulfate, Testosterone, and Estradiol Levels in Middle Aged Men and Postmenopausal Women: A Diet-Controlled Intervention Study," *Alcoholism: Clinical and Experimental Research* 28 (2004): 780–785.

4. J. M. Cohen et al., "Therapeutic Intervention for Chronic Prostatitis/Chronic Pelvic Pain Syndrome (CP/CPPS): A Systematic Review and Meta-analysis," *PLoS One* 7, no. 8 (2012): e41941, doi: 10.1371/journal.pone.0041941.

5. D. A. Tripp et al., "A Survey of Cannabis Use and Self-Reported Benefit in Men with CP/CPPS," *Canadian Urological Association Journal* 8, no. 11 (2014): E901–E905.

6. A. Herati and R. M. Modwin, "Alternative Therapies in the Management of Chronic Prostatitis/Chronic Pelvic Pain Syndrome," *World Journal of Urology* 31, no. 4 (2013): 761–766, doi: 10.1007/s00345-013-1097-0.

7. U.S. Preventive Services Task Force, "Screening for Prostate Cancer: US Preventive Services Task Force Recommendation Statement," *Journal of the American Medical Association* 319, no. 18 (2018): 1901–1913, doi:10.1001/jama.2018.3710.

10

How to Prevent Cancer

Men fear cancer. That's understandable. But the good news is that the risk of many cancers can be significantly reduced through the healthy habits we discuss in this book. In fact, the three most common cancers in men, prostate, lung, and colon—which account for over half of all cancers in men—have been found to have many modifiable risk factors. Overall, 90–95 percent of cancers are the direct result of dietary and other lifestyle factors, including obesity, lack of physical activity, and smoking. Obesity alone accounts for 14 percent of all cancers in men, while poor dietary choices over the long term (high intakes of meat, fat, and processed foods) account for one-third of the risk of cancers in general and 75 percent of the risk of colon and prostate cancer. Of course, for lung cancer, tobacco accounts for 84 percent of the risk.[1]

Men are twice as likely as women to die from cancers due to *preventable* lifestyle factors such as obesity, lack of physical activity, and smoking, according to the World Health Organization.

There is such substantial evidence about the power of lifestyle to prevent cancer that the American Cancer Society has released guidelines on nutrition and physical activity as they relate to cancer prevention (see Box 10.1). They are a great place to start in your quest to prevent cancer.

This chapter will focus on prevention. The treatment of cancer is complicated and best handled with an aggressive approach, with proven modern Western treatments leading the way. There is much good news in cancer treatment—precision medicine techniques can target specific cancers based on an individual's particular cancer genetics, leading to efficacious treatments with minimal side effects—but I will leave that to the specialists. Integrative medicine, which lies at the heart of this book, can play an important role in cancer treatment, in that the many tools we discuss for prevention and optimal health can be used alongside modern Western treatments, especially to mitigate toxicity of chemo and radiation treatments and to prevent recurrence. Large bodies of evidence support the use of complementary therapies along with standard cancer treatments such as surgery, radiation, and chemotherapy.

JIM: FAMILY HISTORY OF CANCER

Jim is fifty-one. His dad had prostate cancer, which was treated successfully. Then his older brother got diagnosed with colon cancer, so he decided to finally have his routine colonoscopy, which had been recommended at age fifty but which he had put off. He thought it would be uncomfortable, but while the prep the night before was annoying (he had to drink a lemonade-flavored laxative that made him go to the bathroom six times, emptying out his colon), the procedure itself was easy—he slept through it with the medication they gave him.

When he woke up after the procedure, the gastroenterologist told him that he had found a polyp and removed it; the tissue would be examined by a pathologist to see if it was cancerous. A few days later, the doctor called Jim to tell him that the polyp was not cancer, but it was precancerous, and so his risk of developing additional polyps was greater than average. The gastroenterologist recommended that Jim have his next colonoscopy in five years instead of the usual ten years.

Those few days waiting for the report about whether or not his polyp was a colon cancer were scary for Jim, given his brother's recent diagnosis. During those few days, he came in to talk with me about his concerns and, in hopes the report would be good, to find out what he could do to make sure he doesn't get colon cancer or any other type of cancer down the road.

Jim's diet is SAD—meaning he eats the standard American diet: chicken, beef, or pork nearly every day, with an occasional fish dish; he usually has some sort of vegetable (corn, potatoes, or maybe green beans or a salad), and he has dessert three or four days a week. He likes his evening snack of frozen yogurt. His weight and height put him at a BMI of 27, which is overweight. He engages in minimal exercise (plays basketball once a week) because he's so busy with work and spending as much time as he can with his partner and their two children, ages twelve and fourteen.

Jim's story is very typical. Many of my patients ask how they can prevent cancer, divulging that they are very worried about getting it because of a friend or relative having a cancer diagnosis or scare. What do I recommend Jim do for prevention of cancer, especially the types for which men are most at risk: prostate, colon, and lung?

First of all, it's important for anyone like Jim who is concerned about having bad genes related to cancer (based on family history or genetic

- Achieve and maintain a healthy weight throughout life.
- Be as lean as possible throughout life without being underweight.
- Avoid excess weight gain at all ages. For those who are currently over weight or obese, losing even a small amount of weight has health benefits and is a good place to start.
- Engage in regular physical activity and limit consumption of high-calorie foods and beverages as key strategies for maintaining a healthy weight.
- Adopt a physically active lifestyle.
- Adults should engage in at least 150 minutes of moderate-intensity activity or 75 minutes of vigorous-intensity activity each week, or an equivalent combination, preferably spread throughout the week.
- Children and adolescents should engage in at least 60 minutes of moderate- or vigorous-intensity activity each day, with vigorous-intensity activity occurring at least three days each week.
- Limit sedentary behavior such as sitting, lying down watching television, or other forms of screen-based entertainment.
- Doing some physical activity above usual activities, no matter what one's level of activity, can have many health benefits.
- Consume a healthy diet, with an emphasis on plant foods.
- Choose foods and beverages in amounts that help achieve and maintain a healthy weight.
- Limit consumption of processed meat and red meat.
- Eat at least 2½ cups of vegetables and fruits each day.
- Choose whole-grain instead of refined-grain products.
- If you drink alcoholic beverages, limit consumption.
- Have no more than two drinks per day (for men).[15]

testing) to know that, according to the National Cancer Institute, only 5–10 percent of all cancers are the direct result of inherited genetic abnormalities. Of course, if you have been found to have particularly risky genetic markers for cancer, it would be prudent to meet with an expert in cancer or genetics to discuss what you can do to either decrease your risk or set up an aggressive screening program.

> Ninety to 95 percent of cancers are *not* related to genetics or family history.

Whether you have such clearly identified risks or not, there are general recommendations that can make a significant difference in your risk of getting cancer. We will start with overall recommendations for all cancers. Afterward I will list some specifics related to those top three cancers in men.

General Cancer Prevention Techniques

1. Lose weight.
2. Exercise.
3. Eat less meat.
4. Eat more plants.
5. Drink 1–2 glasses of wine (or other alcoholic drink) a day, if appropriate for you.
6. Drink green tea.
7. Socialize on a regular basis.
8. Consider taking nutritional supplements.

1. Lose Weight

Being overweight is a risk factor for many cancers, especially of the colon and prostate, and 70 percent of men in the United States are overweight or obese. In fact, people who are overweight have about twice the risk of cancer of the esophagus, stomach, kidney, and liver. Being overweight increases the risk of other cancers as well (pancreas, gallbladder, colon, and thyroid). And being overweight is not just a risk for development of cancer; it also contributes to dying from cancer. Being of normal weight reduces the risk of dying from cancer by 23 percent compared to being overweight.[2]

⟋ It's not clear what exactly the correlation is between weight and cancer. It could be that obesity contributes to low levels of chronic inflammation; it could be because fat (adipose) tissue is hormonally active; or it could be because being overweight is associated with insulin resistance, which contributes to higher levels of growth hormone and of a hormone called leptin, both of which cause cell proliferation (excess cell growth, which is ultimately what cancer is). But one of the more recent realizations about the link between obesity and cancer involves a receptor on cells for mTOR. mTOR stands for mammalian target of rapamycin, but the actual name is not what's important. mTOR levels rise when food is plentiful, encouraging growth of tissue and discouraging the natural process of clearing out old cells and general detoxification activity (called autophagy). It is good for muscle growth to have surges in mTOR, but when mTOR levels stay high (because of excess food intake and excess fat), there is insufficient clearance of damaged cells (some of which could be precancerous) and unregulated growth—the definition of cancer. This is one reason there is very active research into the potential impact of intermittent fasting not only on weight loss but also on decreasing cancer risk. We know that caloric restriction is one of the most proven antiaging interventions, and its contribution to decreasing cancer risk through the decrease in mTOR may be one reason for that.[3]

2. Exercise

Moderate physical activity decreases cancer risk, especially of the colon. Exercising moderately for two and a half hours a week or more strenuously for an hour and fifteen minutes a week has a sizable impact on risk. Moderate exercise can include taking the stairs instead of the elevator, walking the dog, and watching TV while on a treadmill or stationary bicycle.

3. Eat Less Animal Protein, Especially Processed Meats

Processed meats (lunch meats, bacon, sausages, hot dogs) have been declared a class 1 carcinogen by the World Health Organization. This means there is convincing evidence that the agent causes cancer. Other class 1 carcinogens are tobacco and asbestos.[4] Would you knowingly expose yourself to those? Processed meats have been cured, salted, smoked, or otherwise preserved in some way, all of which cause the meat to have more nitrites. These nitrites turn into N-nitroso compounds, which are compounds also found in smokers and people exposed to environmental chemicals that are proven to be linked with cancer.

Many studies have shown that meat in general increases risk of cancer. The Health Professionals Follow-Up Study actually quantified the mortality risk from eating red meat: a one-serving-per-day increase in red meat increased all-cause mortality by 13 percent for unprocessed meat and 20 percent for processed meat such as bacon and cold cuts.[5] It was not entirely clear in this study whether the increased risk was from meat itself or if those who ate more red meat were also more likely to eat fatty foods in general or exercise less, thereby confounding the effects of meat on cancer risk. But the China Study, a large study of diet and its effect on cancer risk among 6,500 people throughout China, found that animal protein was directly correlated with the risk of cancer. Dairy was also found to be associated with cancer risk. The researchers even found that cancer growth in animals could be turned on and off according to the amount of milk protein (casein) consumed.

4. Eat More Plants

Increased fruit and vegetable consumption is associated with lower risk of cancer, especially lung and colon cancers. The cruciferous vegetables, such as cauliflower and broccoli, are especially proven to have anticancer properties. In general, vegetarian diets are associated with decreased risk of cancer, but it is not all-or-nothing. First of all, fish consumption doesn't increase cancer (especially if the fish is wild-caught), and poultry has not been found to have the same cancer associations that red meat has. Generally, the more vegetarian, the better, but it doesn't have to be 100 percent.

In fact, men who stick to a Mediterranean diet (which is not a vegetarian diet, but includes less meat than the standard American diet) have been found to have a 21 percent reduction in cancer risk.[6] As has been discussed, this style of diet is characterized by large amounts of nuts, fruits, vegetables, legumes, whole grains, fish, and olive oil and moderate amounts of meat and red wine, where the wine is largely drunk with meals. The high amounts of omega-3 fatty acids are known to decrease inflammation and to be cancer-protective.

5. Drink One to Two Glasses of Wine a Day

There is a sweet spot when it comes to alcohol consumption and cancer. One to two servings of alcohol a day (each serving is a 6-ounce glass of wine, a 12-ounce beer, or a 1½-ounce shot of hard liquor) seems to be protective; but there is a slightly higher risk of various cancers with no alcohol intake and with greater than an average of two drinks per day.

6. Drink Green Tea

Powerful antioxidants in green tea, called polyphenols, can exert a protective effect, especially in helping to prevent prostate cancer. The research is so compelling that green tea extracts are being studied in the treatment of cancer.

7. Socialization

Belonging to social groups has been shown to increase life span in people diagnosed with cancer.

We've already mentioned the Ornish Reversal program in Chapter 8, on heart health. But the program has also been shown to slow the progression of prostate cancer. One of the most important features of this program is its emphasis on social support: participants engage in group exercise, learn stress management techniques in a group setting, and share about their experiences.

8. Consider Taking Supplements

A meta-analysis of fourteen studies testing a variety of supplements, including vitamin E, vitamin C, zinc, selenium, beta-carotene, and a general multivitamin, did not show that these supplements had any effect on the incidence of prostate cancer or its severity.[7] Another review of studies looking at vitamins C and E did not show that these nutrients had an impact on general cancer risk.[8] But some other supplements have shown more of an effect on risk of cancer.

Curcumin is the main active ingredient in turmeric, used for centuries as a medicinal herb and in foods as a spice, especially in Indian food. It is known to have potent anti-inflammatory effects. Several studies have also shown it to have anti-cancer effects as well, but it is poorly absorbed unless taken with piperine (found in black pepper).[9] So when cooking with turmeric, be sure to add a little pepper, and when shopping for a supplement with curcumin, be sure it also has piperine.

What about folate? There had been studies showing a possible preventive effect of folic acid on prostate cancer. Then a study was published in 2006 showing that supplementation with folic acid actually *increased* prostate cancer risk. These seemingly conflicting studies have since been further analyzed, and it appears that natural folate (aka vitamin B_9), found in foods such as dark leafy greens, asparagus, broccoli, and beans, may help to prevent prostate cancer, while artificial folic acid, which must be converted in the body to active folate, may increase the risk. So look for supplements with folate, as opposed to folic acid.

Vitamin D may help to decrease the risk of colon cancer. A review of studies looking at populations and their vitamin D intake or blood levels of vitamin D did show that more vitamin D was associated with lower colon cancer risk.[10] Studies have tried to confirm that taking vitamin D actually lowers risk, but those have not been so conclusive.

There are other supplements that are potentially helpful in preventing cancer or even slowing the growth of cancer, such as medicinal mushrooms, fish oil, chlorella, and indole-3-carbinol. I haven't seen strong enough evidence yet to strongly recommend them, but these are all worth keeping an eye on for studies proving their benefit.

TED: THE CANCER GENE

Ted's father has prostate cancer, so he came in for a check of his own prostate. In asking him about his family history, I learned that his maternal aunt had had ovarian cancer and his maternal grandmother had had breast cancer. All of these cancers are linked, in that they are all related to hormones, and there's a genetic variant that can increase the risk for any of these three cancers. So when we found that Ted's prostate was normal at this time, I thought it was worth discussing with Ted whether he wanted to be tested for the genes that are associated with such hormonally responsive cancers, BRCA1 and BRCA2. Men with the BRCA2 gene have almost a ninefold higher risk of prostate cancer, and men with the BRCA1 gene have a risk that's almost four times higher.

Whether such genetic testing is right for someone is a highly personal decision. In Ted's case, would he want to know if he was at such increased risk? If he found out he carried one of these genes, would it spur him to make changes in habits that might help protect him? Would he be motivated to get more frequent screening? Or would it just keep him up at night, worrying?

Genetic Testing

If you are considering getting tested to see whether you carry any genes that might increase your risk of cancer, it is important to think about how the results will impact your life. What would you do if you found you do have genes that confer higher risk for the development of cancer? Perhaps you would be more likely to follow a vegan diet or opt for more aggressive screening if you knew you were at higher risk. Some people would just end up feeling highly anxious all the time, worrying that they might get cancer. There is no right or wrong about getting genetic testing done—it is a personal decision that depends on your own nature.

Ted ended up feeling that "knowledge is power" and opted for the test. It did show he had the BRCA2 gene. While this was very concerning, it spurred him to dramatically cut down on his consumption of bacon and hot dogs and to increase his exercise. He also added foods rich in lycopene to his diet and lost weight. Equally important, he was able to discuss with his wife the importance of having their daughter's genetic testing done, to see if she needed to start early screening for breast cancer.

Prostate Cancer Prevention

Prostate cancer is the most common cancer found in men, accounting for 25 percent of all cancer diagnoses. Even though it is the second most common cause of cancer deaths in men, only a small percent of those diagnosed with the disease die of it. Most men with prostate cancer will die *with* the disease, not *from* the disease—meaning that while the statistic that one in seven men will develop prostate cancer in his lifetime is frightening, the fact is that the vast majority have very early-stage cancers that either don't ever need treatment or are curable. This is not to minimize the tragedy of advanced prostate cancer and its impact on the lives of many men; I only hope to decrease anxiety over a possible initial diagnosis. As Table 10.1 shows, there are proportionately far fewer deaths from prostate cancer than from other leading cancers in men.

In terms of prevention of prostate cancer, it's important to keep in mind that the main risk factors are age (95 percent of all cases are in men age fifty or over), African ancestry, and family history. Obesity, eating a diet high in meat or dairy, and smoking all increase the chance of prostate cancer being more aggressive, but they may not increase the actual risk of getting prostate cancer.

Screening for prostate cancer is controversial, because there is conflicting data on the usefulness of the main blood test used for screening, the prostate-specific antigen (PSA) test. I suggest you ask your primary care provider about the best screening for you. Newer tests, including the free-PSA blood test, the prostate health index (PHI), and prostate MRIs, have improved the ability to predict whether or not cancer is present and to direct biopsies more specifically. This will hopefully improve the ability to detect early cancers and to avoid unnecessary biopsies in men who have elevated PSAs but no cancer.

Table 10.1 Cancers in Men per Year

	New Cases	Deaths
All Cancers	822,000	300,000
Prostate	241,000	33,000
Lung	115,000	86,000
Colon	72,000	23,000

The best ways to avoid aggressive prostate cancer are as follows:

1. Don't smoke. Smoking increases the risk of dying from prostate cancer: a meta-analysis of twenty-four studies confirmed that the heaviest smokers had up to 30 percent greater risk of death from prostate cancer.[11]
2. Eat less red meat. Men who eat the most red meat have higher risks for prostate cancer, especially advanced prostate cancer that is harder to treat and more aggressive.
3. Maintain a healthy weight. There is a strong link between obesity and death from prostate cancer.
4. Eat more plant foods. Higher vegetable intake, especially cruciferous vegetables like broccoli, cauliflower, and Brussels sprouts, is associated with decreased prostate cancer risk.
5. Eat foods with lycopene. Lycopene is a carotenoid pigment found in red foods, like tomatoes. It is especially well absorbed when tomatoes are cooked and mixed with oil (such as in a nice, healthy red sauce with olive oil). While the evidence is somewhat conflicting, several studies have shown a protective benefit from this antioxidant.
6. Drink pomegranate juice. This juice is rich in polyphenols, and drinking 8 ounces a day has been shown to decrease recurrence of prostate cancer (in one small industry-sponsored study) and to slow progression of prostate cancer (in another study not funded by industry).[12,13] Research has shown that pomegranate juice can reduce the growth of prostate cancer cells in the lab. Just make sure you are drinking 100 percent pure pomegranate juice, without added sugar.
7. Have your vitamin D level checked. Low levels of 1,25-hydroxy-vitamin D (less than 30 ng/mL) are associated with an increased risk for many problems, including prostate cancer. If your level is low, it is prudent to supplement with vitamin D_3 to increase your level. Ask a medical provider how much you should take.

Colon Cancer Prevention

Colon cancer is the third-leading cause of cancer in men and is more common in men than women. Most cancers of the colon start as polyps, which take ten to fifteen years to grow into cancers. So the best way to avoid colon cancer is to have routine screening colonoscopy exams to look for any polyps.

Colon cancer is 60 percent more common in Western countries, where our diet is more likely due to include processed and other unhealthy foods. It makes sense that dietary changes are the most powerful way to prevent colon cancer, since the colon is so intimately connected with what we eat.

Reducing colon cancer risk involves the following:

1. Eat more fiber. Increased fiber contributes directly to a lower risk of colon cancer, according to multiple studies and a large meta-analysis.[14] The amount of fiber recommended to avoid colon cancer is 30 grams or more a day.
2. Increase your consumption of omega-3 fatty acids (fish oil). Studies have found large differences in rates of colon cancer depending on how much fish is consumed (the more fish, the less risk). Of course, be wary of the larger fish (tuna, halibut, shark), which are more likely to have a higher mercury content.
3. Eat less red and processed meat. As has been mentioned before, processed meat (sausage, lunch meat, bacon) is considered a carcinogen by the World Health Organization. Even unprocessed red meat increases risk of colon cancer, partly in and of itself and partly from the heterocyclic amines and polycyclic hydrocarbons that are formed when meat is fried or grilled.
4. Eat garlic. Several studies show that high consumption of garlic decreases the risk for colon cancer.
5. Maintain a healthy weight. There it is again—obesity contributes to colon cancer risk.
6. Take vitamin D. Just as low vitamin D levels are correlated with increased risk for prostate cancer, it is the same for cancer of the colon. Taking vitamin D_3 can help get your blood levels of this vitamin above 50 ng/ml, with the ideal level being between 50 and 100 ng/dL.

Lung Cancer Prevention

Lung cancer is the second most common cancer and the leading cause of cancer deaths in the United States, accounting for 28 percent of all cancer-related deaths and 13 percent of all cancer diagnoses in men. The good news is that the incidence has been declining since the 1980s due to a drop in tobacco use.

How can you minimize your risk of getting lung cancer?

1. Don't smoke or be around people who smoke. Cigarette smoking is by far the strongest risk factor for lung cancer; 90 percent of lung cancers are the result of tobacco use, and the risk of a smoker developing lung cancer is twenty-five times greater than that of a non-smoker. Secondhand smoke is also a factor, causing more than 7,000 deaths per year from lung cancer.
2. Avoid exposure to other environmental carcinogens as much as possible. Exposure to radon, asbestos, heavy metals, air pollution, radiation, and diesel exhaust also contribute to the risk of getting lung cancer. Minimizing exposure or wearing proper masks when working with known toxic chemicals will help reduce risk.
3. Consider supplements. If you are particularly concerned about your risk for lung cancer based on a personal history of smoking or toxin exposure, consider supplements that can improve your body's antioxidative capacity, such as curcumin, discussed earlier in this chapter. Curcumin has anti-inflammatory, antioxidant, and immune-boosting effects. It even has been shown to decrease the growth of new blood vessels that can contribute to tumor growth. Just remember that it needs to be taken with black pepper to improve its absorption.

The Bottom Line

All in all, you do have more control over your likelihood of getting cancer than you might think. Even if you have unfavorable genes, your lifestyle has a great impact on your individual risk of developing cancer. The most common cancers in men, prostate, lung, and colon, are among those that are most strongly linked with poor diet, excess weight, exposures to toxins, and lack of exercise. Therefore they are the cancers you can be most active in preventing.

Questions to Ask Your Doctor

1. What's the best way for me to be checked for prostate cancer?
2. Do I really need a prostate biopsy? (If you have an elevated PSA, ask about a free PSA test, the prostate health index, and/or prostate MRI before agreeing to a biopsy.)
3. At what age should I have my first colonoscopy?
4. What's the healthiest weight for me?

Notes

1. P. Anand et al., "Cancer Is a Preventable Disease That Requires Major Lifestyle Changes," *Pharmaceutical Research* 25, no. 9 (2008): 2097–2116, doi: 10.1007/s11095-008-9661-9.

2. D. C. Whiteman and L. F. Wilson, "The Fractions of Cancer Attributable to Modifiable Factors: A Global Review," *Cancer Epidemiology* 44 (2016): 203-221, doi: 10.1016/j.canep.2016.06.013.

3. D. L. Roberts, C. Dive, and A. G. Renehan, "Biological Mechanisms Linking Obesity and Cancer Risk: New Perspectives," *Annual Review of Medicine* 61 (2010): 301–316, doi: 10.1146/annurev.med.080708.082713.

4. World Health Organization, "Q&A on the Carcinogenicity of the Consumption of Red Meat and Processed Meat," October 2015, http://www.who.int/features/qa/cancer-red-meat/en.

5. A. Pan et al., "Red Meat Consumption and Mortality: Results from Two Prospective Cohort Studies," *Archives of Internal Medicine* 172, no. 7 (2012): 555–563, doi:10.1001/archinternmed.2011.2287.

6. L. Verbene et al., "Association Between the Mediterranean Diet and Cancer Risk: A Review of Observational Studies," *Nutrition and Cancer* 62, no. 7 (2010): 860–870, doi: 10.1080/01635581.2010.509834.

7. J. Straton and M. Godwin, "The Effect of Supplemental Vitamins and Minerals on the Development of Prostate Cancer: Systematic Review and Meta Analysis," *Family Practice* 28, no. 3 (2011): 243–252, doi: 10.1093/fampra/cmq115.

8. I. Coulter et al., *Effect of the Supplemental Use of Antioxidants Vitamin C, Vitamin E, and Coenzyme Q10 for the Prevention and Treatment of Cancer*, Evidence Reports/Technology Assessments no. 75 (Rockville, MD: Agency for Healthcare Research and Quality, 2003), https://www.ncbi.nlm.nih.gov/books/NBK36859.

9. W. Park et al., "New Perspectives of Curcumin in Cancer Prevention," *Cancer Prevention Research* 6, no. 5 (2013): 387–400, doi:10.1158/1940-6207.CAPR-12-0410.

10. Y. Ma et al., "Association Between Vitamin D and Risk of Colorectal Cancer: A Systematic Review of Prospective Studies," *Journal of Clinical Oncology* 29, no. 28 (2011): 3775–3782, doi: 10.1200/JCO.2011.35.7566.

11. Lora A. Plaskon et al., "Cigarette Smoking and Risk of Prostate Cancer in Middle-Aged Men," *Cancer Epidemiology, Biomarkers, and Prevention* 12, no. 7 (2003): 604–609.

12. C. J. Paller et al., "A Randomized Phase II Study of Pomegranate Extract for Men with Rising PSA Following Initial Therapy for Localized Prostate

Cancer," *Prostate Cancer and Prostatic Diseases* 16 (2013): 50, doi: 10.1038/pcan.2012.20.

13. A. J. Pantuck et al., "Phase II Study of Pomegranate Juice for Men with Rising PSA Following Surgery or Radiation for Prostate Cancer," *Clinical Cancer Research* 12, no. 13 (2006): 4018–4026, doi: 10.1158/1078-0432.CCR-05-2290.

14. Aune Dagfinn et al., "Dietary Fibre, Whole Grains, and Risk of Colorectal Cancer: Systematic Review and Dose-Response Meta-Analysis of Prospective Studies," *BMJ* 343 (2011): d6617, doi: 10.1136/bmj.d6617.

15. L. H. Kushi et al., "American Cancer Society Guidelines on Nutrition and Physical Activity for Cancer Prevention: Reducing the Risk of Cancer with Healthy Food Choices and Physical Activity," *CA: A Cancer Journal for Clinicians* 62, no. 1 (2012): 30–67, doi: 10.3322/caac.20140.

Resources

The Movember Foundation has great resources about cancer in men: https://us.movember.com.

The China Study, by T. Colin Campbell with Thomas M. Campbell II (Dallas, TX: BenBella Books, 2016), and the documentary based on this book, *Forks over Knives*, are both about one of the largest studies to date showing the link between eating meat and cancer.

Jack M., "Prostate Cancer Was My Doorway into Vibrant Health and an Expansive and Happy Life," Ornish Living, https://www.ornish.com/zine/prostate-cancer-doorway-vibrant-health-expansive-happy-life.

Information from the American Cancer Society on genetic testing for cancer: https://www.cancer.org/cancer/cancer-causes/genetics/understanding-genetic-testing-for-cancer.html.

World Health Organization FAQs about meat being labeled a carcinogen: http://www.who.int/features/qa/cancer-red-meat/en.

11

Optimal Sexual Health

This may be the first chapter of this book that you turned to, because sexual issues are one of the most common health problems reported by men. Whether it's low libido, erectile dysfunction, or premature ejaculation, it may be due to hormonal issues, such as low testosterone, but not necessarily. So this chapter will discuss hormone replacement with testosterone, but it will also cover other causes of sexual issues along with non-hormonal treatments for these problems.

Erectile Dysfunction (ED)

ED is one of the common issues men face, as evidenced by the popularity of Viagra, Cialis, Levitra, and the other ED medications. ED is not only a problem for older men: approximately 20 percent of men under the age of forty-nine suffer from at least moderate erectile dysfunction.

ED can be caused by a multitude of issues, from poor blood flow to a lack of the right neurotransmitters, the nervous system chemicals that must be turned on in order to stimulate the dilation of arteries, allowing more blood flow to create and maintain an erection.[1] What can cause issues with blood flow or neurotransmitters? General medical issues such as hypertension, obesity, high cholesterol, and diabetes all contribute to plaque in arteries all over the body (atherosclerosis), which can mean less blood flow to the penis as well. Neurotransmitter release is affected by perceived stress, anxiety, mood, diet, and medications, all of which can impact ED. Box 11.1 lists the most common risk factors for erectile dysfunction.

Box 11.1 Risk Factors for ED

Age

Cardiovascular disease

Tobacco smoking

Diabetes

Hormonal disorders, such as low thyroid, low testosterone, high prolactin, high estrogen

High cholesterol

Hypertension

Obesity

Psychological issues, such as stress, anxiety, depression, history of sexual abuse, relationship problems

Sedentary lifestyle

Medications

Antihistamines

Benzodiazepines (Xanax [alprazolam], Klonopin [clonazepam], Valium [diazepam])

Beta blockers (Toprol [metoprolol], Tenormin [atenolol])

SSRIs (Prozac [fluoxetine], Lexapro [escitalopram], Celexa [citalopram], Zoloft [sertraline], Paxil [paroxetine])

Narcotic pain medications (Vicodin [hydrocodone], Percocet [oxycodone])

Illicit drugs

Alcohol

When erections are not what they used to be, the first approach is to look at what lifestyle factors can be improved, such as quitting smoking, increasing exercise, or losing weight. Next, treatment of medical issues such as high blood pressure, high cholesterol, and diabetes should be optimized. Hormone levels should be checked, and any abnormalities treated. It is also prudent to check for overall atherosclerosis in a man who complains of ED, as this may be the first sign of a systemic problem with blockage of arteries not only in the penis but also around the heart or in the arteries leading to the brain, increasing the risk of heart attack or stroke. Next, a review of drugs and alcohol taken should be done to make sure there is no contribution here. Narcotic pain medications, marijuana, stimulants like Adderall, alcohol, and antihistamines (used to treat indigestion or allergies) can interfere with erections.

In terms of treatment for ED, most men know about medications like Viagra and Cialis (phosphodiesterase (PDE5)-inhibitors). These are effective but can have side effects and are very costly. So, what else can be done for ED? While there are supplements that can help, this is one condition requiring a true mind-body approach. If any of the psychological issues listed in Box 11.1 (depression, anxiety, relationship issues, etc.) are present—and there often is something that rings true in this list for most men with ED—no amount of medical treatment will help if those issues aren't addressed. This can be with a therapist solo, in couples counseling, or even with an expert in trauma, if needed. Mindfulness relaxation can be a big benefit to those with anxiety, and there are many classes and apps that can help with that; the resources at the end of the chapter list some, and more are discussed in Chapter 6, on managing stress. But ignoring any psychological contribution to ED will undermine your other efforts.

Supplements

There are several supplements that have been shown to be helpful in treating ED. Before I list the most useful ones, a word of warning: ED is one of the most common reasons men seek out nutritional supplements. The PDE5-inhibitor medications are very expensive, and many men are desperate for help improving the quality of their erections. There are a lot of unscrupulous companies and poor-quality supplements out there, so I highly recommend you ask your medical provider for help choosing legitimate, safe, and high-quality supplements. As was discussed in Chapter 4, supplements are not closely regulated, and the sexual performance category is particularly rife with adulterated supplements or those that don't contain the ingredients they say they do. The FDA has found that many products marketed for ED either contain contaminants, are mislabeled, or even contain potentially dangerous ingredients. Listed in Table 11.1 are a few botanicals and other supplements that do have sufficient evidence of their usefulness for ED, but make sure the brand you buy is a good-quality one.[2]

Other Modalities

Acupuncture

Acupuncture can be of benefit to men suffering from ED. It may be coupled with Chinese herbs, such as *Panax ginseng*, depending on the recommendation of the Chinese medical practitioner. Acupuncture can help the flow of the chi essence in the body, which can correlate with improvements in blood and energy flow in general.

Lifestyle

As mentioned, there is a strong correlation between lifestyle-associated chronic diseases, such as obesity, diabetes, and hypertension, and ED. In fact, because such diseases contribute to blockages of the arteries, ED may be a manifestation of one of the underlying diseases caused by poor lifestyle choices. ED can be a symptom of cardiovascular disease in general, appearing two to three years before any other symptoms such as hypertension or symptoms of coronary artery disease like chest pain or shortness of breath. This makes it especially important to seek advice from your practitioner if you have ED, as the workup for this problem can identify early, and possibly reversible, signs of systemic cardiovascular disease.

No particular diet or exercise routine can be recommended for ED specifically, but anything that helps heart disease, such as the Mediterranean or anti-inflammatory diet and regular exercise, can help treat or prevent ED.

PHIL: PREMATURE EJACULATION

Phil came to me with a problem he had never discussed with any medical provider before: he wasn't able to prevent himself from ejaculating longer than a minute or so during intercourse. This was frustrating for him and for his partner, so he finally sheepishly asked me if there was anything he could do about it. I was so glad he brought it up! Doctors, even specialists in men's health, typically don't think to ask about the problem of premature ejaculation (PE), even though it is very common, can cause terrible distress, and can even sabotage relationships. And there are some things men can do to improve the problem.

We talked about some easy quick things to try, such as using a little prescription lidocaine gel mixed with lubricant that he could apply topically before putting on a condom. I also suggested he try pulling out before getting close to orgasm (even if it was after one minute) to pinch the head of his penis sharply or slap his own inner thigh sharply before reinserting. We also talked about other options such as medications and mind-body techniques.

In the end, he decided to use an antidepressant medication, Prozac (fluoxetine), to be taken only on days when he planned to have intercourse, and to start a mindfulness practice using an app on his smartphone. When he was alone, he practiced the mental focus he was learning during masturbation, when he would stop himself before getting close to orgasm and allow his sexual excitement to simmer down before starting again. In this way, he was able to prolong his time before ejaculating on his own and during intercourse with his partner.

Table 11.1 Supplements Useful in Treating ED

Supplement	Dose	Comments
Yohimbine	5–10 mg 3 times daily	Yohimbine is derived from the bark of a tree native to central and western Africa. It has been used for decades for ED, with some success. Especially when combined with L-arginine, it can dilate blood vessels, allowing for greater blood flow, which facilitates achieving and maintaining erections. Yohimbine can lower blood pressure and increase heart rate, so take caution with its use if you have low blood pressure or are taking nitrates for your heart or monoamine oxidase inhibitor medications for depression (rarely used these days).
L-arginine	1,000–2,000 mg 3 times daily when used alone, or 500 mg 2 or 3 times daily when combined with yohimbine or pycnogenol	Converted by the body into nitric oxide, which dilates small arteries. When combined with yohimbine or with another botanical, pycnogenol (from pine bark), it can dramatically improve ED.
Panax ginseng (Korean red ginseng)	1,800–3,000 mg daily	A meta-analysis of seven studies has shown that *Panax ginseng* can be helpful.[8] (Note that there are different herbs called ginseng; make sure you select *Panax ginseng*.) Side effects are rare but can include insomnia. There is a topical formulation that can also be helpful.

Table 11.1 continued

Supplement	Dose	Comments
Maca	500–1,000 mg 2 or 3 times daily	Maca, from the root of a plant that grows mostly in the Andes, is effective against lower libido and delayed ejaculation. It was even found to reverse some of the sexual side effects caused by SSRI antidepressants.[9]
Gingko biloba	240 mg daily	Gingko can cause mild gastrointestinal upset in some, but it can also counter some of the sexual side effects of SSRI antidepressants. Some reports show it also helps cognition and memory.
DHEA	25–50 mg daily	Prohormone made in the adrenal glands that decreases with age and with chronic stress. Taking DHEA can help ED in men who have low DHEA levels (best measured as DHEA sulfate level).

Premature Ejaculation (PE)

Up to 20 percent of men report premature ejaculation (so most likely many more actually experience it but don't report it), with many more feeling that they would rather be able to control ejaculation better. This is a significant source of stress for the man and for his partner and is associated with anxiety and depression, especially when it means that intercourse usually doesn't last longer than a minute or two.

There are a few medications that can help with PE, such as SSRI antidepressants, including Prozac, Zoloft (sertraline), Lexapro (escitalopram), Celexa (citalopram), and Paxil (paroxetine). These so reliably cause a delay in ejaculation that they can be used for treatment for PE on an as-needed basis. Applying topical lidocaine gel (an anesthetic) to the penis, when used along with a condom to prevent causing numbness to the partner, can be helpful. As many as 50 percent of men with PE also have ED, so we will often use PDE-5 inhibitors, such as sildenafil, along with fluoxetine.

The pain medication Ultram (tramadol) has also been found to be helpful for PE, especially when used sporadically. A small study of 60 patients in India found that 100 mg of tramadol increased time to ejaculation during intercourse (from 1 minute to about 4 minutes).[3]

There are nonpharmaceutical approaches to this condition as well. Yoga has been found to be very helpful, perhaps because it allows for greater control over the body and more relaxation. Mindfulness practice can help control over thoughts and over the body's level of excitement. Other mind-body interventions such as hypnosis can be powerful treatments for PE. Simple maneuvers such as sharply and very briefly pinching the head of the penis or slapping the inner thigh when stimulation rises too quickly can help to pull excitement back from approaching the point of no return. Acupuncture and Chinese herbs can be helpful as well.

Key Behaviors to Minimize or Alleviate ED and PE

For Erectile Dysfunction
- Exercise.
- Eat a Mediterranean diet.
- Employ stress reduction techniques.
- Avoid tobacco.
- Decrease alcohol consumption.
- Maintain a normal weight.
- Avoid heating or storing foods in plastics (to decrease exposure to hormone-disrupting substances).
- Try mindfulness apps (Headspace, Calm, Insight Timer, 10% Happier; see Chapter 6).

Premature Ejaculation

- Try yoga.
- Use SSRI medications as needed.
- Physical maneuvers can temporarily decrease arousal.
- Hypnotherapy can be effective.

Testosterone

Testosterone (T) deficiency, in which the level of T falls below what is considered normal for men of that age, affects approximately 30 percent of men between forty and seventy-nine years old. There is a strong correlation between low T and preventable lifestyle-related diseases such as obesity, diabetes, hypertension, and metabolic syndrome, so treating these conditions if they're present—and taking steps to prevent them—goes a long way toward improving the level of testosterone.

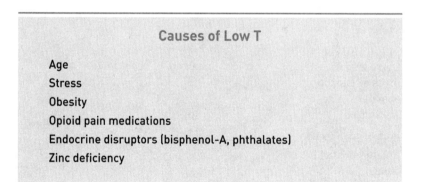

Causes of Low T

Age
Stress
Obesity
Opioid pain medications
Endocrine disruptors (bisphenol-A, phthalates)
Zinc deficiency

Stress is probably the most common cause of low T, because when the body perceives stress, whether due to illness, injury, emotional stress, or anxiety, cellular pathways get stimulated that lead to a blunted drive for sex and reproduction and an increase in survival-mode fight-or-flight-type activities. When you are chronically stressed and not managing it well, your

Optimal Sexual Health

body stays in ready-to-respond mode, which is quite the opposite of relaxed and sexual. The impact is measurable through increases in stress hormones like cortisol and adrenaline (epinephrine) and decreases in testosterone and another male hormone involved in sex drive, DHEA.

All of these factors lower testosterone levels in men of any age, but I would argue that even the "normal" testosterone decline that happens with age, starting around thirty-five—what can be called andropause—may warrant treatment if it is accompanied by symptoms, which can be physical, psychological, and/or sexual. Table 11.2 shows these symptoms of low T. If you have any of them, it is worth getting your T levels checked.

Finding out your level is important, not only so that you and your doctor can decide on the best ways to alleviate sexual symptoms but also because low T is actually dangerous. In fact, several studies have shown that low testosterone is associated with an increase in mortality in men over forty.

Table 11.2 Symptoms of Low Testosterone

Physical	Sexual	Psychological
Decreased muscle mass or inability to gain muscle despite working out	Erectile dysfunction	Low general energy
Increased body fat	Low libido	Mild depression
Enlargement of breast tissue	Difficulty achieving orgasm	Memory or concentration issues
Fatigue	Decreased morning erections	
Anemia		
Decreased bone density		

Conditions Associated with Low T

- Increased mortality
- Increased risk for heart attack and stroke
- Bone loss

Many doctors don't even recognize that the treatment of low T can be as important for overall health and longevity as the treatment of high cholesterol or low vitamin D.[4] One major study showed that among men with the lowest levels of testosterone, for every 173 ng/dL increase in serum T, keeping it in the normal range, there was a 21 percent lower risk of death (the normal range for T is approximately 300–1,000 ng/dL).[5] In fact, treating low T with testosterone replacement has been shown not only to reduce risk of mortality but also to improve libido, sexual function, bone strength, muscle strength, and exercise capacity. The use of testosterone replacement has been shown to increase serum testosterone to bring it back to normal levels, improve libido, reduce erectile dysfunction, improve overall sexual function, increase energy, improve mood, increase bone mineral density, decrease body fat mass, and increase lean body muscle mass.

What are the options for treating low testosterone? If the level is truly low and there are symptoms to match, I generally recommend true testosterone replacement therapy. For this, there are various testosterone preparations available; see Table 11.3 for a list.

There are other forms of testosterone that some men use, such as anabolic steroids, that are specifically formulated to target muscle growth. These are often not legal in the United States and are unregulated. I don't recommend these, as what is sold may be impure, adulterated, or inconsistent from bottle to bottle. And they can have many undesirable side effects, especially with long-term use. If you are looking for more muscle growth, it is best to see if you actually have low testosterone levels. If you do, prescription T using any of the formulations listed in the table can definitely help build muscle mass. If your levels are normal, taking more T is likely to produce more side effects than benefits.

Table 11.3 Testosterone Replacement Therapy Options

How used	Frequency	Advantages	Disadvantages
Intramuscular T injection	Once or twice a week	Long-acting, relatively inexpensive if self-administered, flexibility of dosing	Requires intramuscular injection (usually in buttock or thigh), creates peaks and troughs in T levels
Intramuscular long-acting T injection	Once a month	Infrequent administration	Large-volume (4 ml) intramuscular injection; risk of fat embolism
Subcutaneous T injection	Once a week	Long-acting, relatively inexpensive if self-administered, flexibility of dosing, ease of administration with subcutaneous injector pen; more stable T levels than intramuscular testosterone	Requires injection, but only under the skin
Topical T gel or cream (on skin, in nose, or under arms, depending on formulation)	TK	Flexible dosing, ease of application, well tolerated	Risk of transfer to a female partner or child by skin-to-skin contact; some men don't achieve much increase in level with topical preparations; some gels have a strong scent

Table 11.3 continued

How used	Frequency	Advantages	Disadvantages
Transdermal T patch	Worn continuously	None	Patch is awkward and can cause contact dermatitis (rash or blister)
T pellets (Testopel) inserted under skin	Every four to six months	Infrequent dosing	Requires surgical incision for insertions; pellets may extrude spontaneously; possible scar formation
Clomid (clomiphene)	TK	Convenience of oral administration; preserves fertility; maintains testicle size	Off-label use for men; not covered by insurance
HCG (human chorionic gonadotropin) subcutaneous injections	TK	Preserves fertility; maintains testicle size; maintains body's own T production	Requires subcutaneous injection

Other Options to Treat Low T

Besides testosterone replacement, there are several other ways to go when treating low T. One pharmaceutical option is off-label use of Clomid (clomiphene), a medication approved to treat infertility in women. Clomiphene increases stimulation of the body's own production of testosterone by affecting the way the hypothalamus and pituitary gland impact testicular production. It has been studied for infertility in men with some success, because testosterone replacement therapy itself should not be used in men actively trying to impregnate a partner.[6] Subcutaneous HCG (human chorionic gonadotropin) has also been used. This hormone is naturally secreted by the pituitary, stimulating testosterone production by the testicles. In men who have low T due to poor pituitary function, treatment with HCG can be helpful.

Another pharmaceutical approach is to block the conversion of testosterone to estrogen, a process that happens naturally via the enzyme aromatase. Blocking this enzyme can increase T while decreasing estradiol, a particularly useful approach for men with both low T and symptoms of estrogen dominance, such as growth of breast tissue or inability to lose fat. Medications such as Arimidex (anastrazole) and Nolvadex (tamoxifen) are used on an off-label basis for this, so it's important to discuss the pros and cons with your doctor, who should closely monitor hormone levels to adjust treatment and prevent side effects. For example, too-low estrogen, even in men, can contribute to rapid loss of bone density, leading to osteopenia or osteoporosis.

Most non-pharmacological approaches to treating low T don't actually raise testosterone. They can help with the symptoms of low T, such as low libido, erectile dysfunction, or low energy, but none directly impact the testosterone level in the body. Instead, some, such as zinc and quercetin, can increase testosterone indirectly by decreasing the body's conversion of testosterone to estrogen. Box 11.2 lists supplements that can help with symptoms of low T.

Addressing causes of low T such as stress or obesity can help to increase T levels as well. If you take narcotic pain medications, discontinuing their use will make a big difference in T level. Positive health behaviors, such as exercise, diet, and avoidance of smoking, are ways to prevent testosterone deficiency, and they correlate significantly with higher testosterone levels over time. And resistance training or high-intensity cardio will raise the body's natural production of testosterone.

Box 11.2 Natural Treatments for Symptoms of Low Testosterone

Panax ginseng, 100–200 mg daily

Maca, 500–1,000 mg 2 or 3 times daily

Tribulus, 250 mg 3 times daily

Horny goat weed, 1,000 mg daily

DHEA, 25–50 mg

Green tea

Zinc (if level is low), 25–50 mg

Quercetin, 400 mg

DHEA, 25–50 mg

Pycnogenol, 50 mg 3 times daily

You may have heard about the use of bioidentical hormones in women, and wonder whether that's an issue for men. It's not, because all testosterone replacement therapy is bioidentical, unlike the hormonal replacement often used for women.

Risks of T Treatment

A few years ago there were several reports of studies showing a risk of heart attack, stroke, or even premature death from T treatment. For the most part, these were based on studies that looked at T in elderly men with preexisting risks for heart problems. There does not seem to be such risks for men under the age of sixty-five without a prior history of heart disease; however, any man initiating testosterone treatment should do so under the care of a medical practitioner who is trained to assess the risks and appropriateness of hormonal therapy and monitor the results.

There are known side effects to testosterone treatment, especially when the dosing drives your level fairly high. The main things to watch for are acne, mood changes (such as becoming more easily agitated), or breast tissue growth (gynecomastia, a result of conversion of extra testosterone to estrogens). A known side effect is increased red blood cell count, a condition that can be dangerous if not treated (usually with phlebotomy, or drawing blood out of your veins), so your blood count should be monitored along with your testosterone level if you are receiving replacement therapy. T treatment does not increase the risk for prostate cancer; this has been shown in multiple studies.[7] However, T can make existing prostate cancer grow, so if you are receiving treatment, you *must* also be screened regularly for prostate cancer. Lastly, because all testosterone therapy (except for treatment with clomiphene or HCG) effectively takes the place of the body's own natural production of T, the testicles, which normally produce testosterone, invariably shrink to some extent. Natural production will come back when T therapy is stopped, with a concomitant return to normal testicle size, but it is something to be aware of. Because of this, therapy with testosterone shouldn't be stopped abruptly, but should be tapered based on discussion with a health provider.

T Measurement

Lastly, a word about how testosterone levels are measured. Most testosterone in the body is bound to protein (albumin or a protein called sex hormone binding globulin), so it's not able to bind to testosterone receptors and have active effects. Therefore, measuring the level of free, unbound testosterone is a better assessment of true hormone status than total testosterone. I recommend starting with a total T level. If this is on the low side, I'd then retest, along with testing for free testosterone and estradiol. At that point a blood count (hemoglobin or hematocrit) and PSA should also be checked as baseline measures. If you're receiving T treatment, your levels should be checked again after four to six weeks and then at least every six months thereafter, including a test of PSA and blood count. Treatment needs to be individualized, so the dose you take may be different from what your friend or gym buddy uses. The goal is alleviating symptoms, and for this the doctor will usually recommend maintaining the total T level in the 500–700 ng/dL range.

The Bottom Line

While sexual issues are common and can be complicated, this chapter offers a few pharmacological, lifestyle, and other options for prevention and treatment of problems ranging from ED to premature ejaculation to low T. Take a look at the resources listed at the end of this chapter. And I always recommend that you discuss with a trusted medical provider any problems that are interfering with your quality of life. Sex is a natural and important part of life and of intimacy, so it is no less of a legitimate concern than other medical issues you would address with your doctor.

Questions to Ask Your Doctor

1. Can you check my T? (If you are feeling low-energy, moody, or depressed, if you can't seem to gain muscle despite working out, or if you have low sex drive, ask your medical provider for a check of testosterone, especially if you are over forty.)
2. What can I do about my low level of testosterone? (If your testosterone is low, ask about all the options for treating it.)
3. What can I do about the decrease in quality of my erections? (If you are having issues maintaining an erection or having as strong an erection as you are used to, look at your diet, physical activity, and level of stress first, before jumping to medications. But talk to your doctor about it, because there may be other reversible causes to check.)
4. Is it okay for me to take the Viagra or ED supplement I ordered online? (Before ordering any pharmaceutical medications or supplements online, ask your own doctor about side effects or possible interactions with other medications you may be taking.)

Notes

1. In order for an erection to happen and be maintained, a cascade of events must happen involving the endocrine (hormonal), nervous, and circulatory systems. The main part of the nervous system involved in erections is the parasympathetic nervous system, which is associated with relaxation. So any emotional or physical stress will interfere on that level. Blood flows through the penile artery, which is relatively small, so any blockage of flow from atherosclerosis may be noticed as less strong erections before any other manifestations arise.
2. Supplements in the United States are not regularly regulated for quality (see Chapter 4).
3. Amil H. Khan and Deepa Rasaily, "Tramadol Use in Premature Ejaculation: Daily vs. Sporadic Treatment," *Indian Journal of Psychological Medicine* 35, no. 3 (2013): 256–259, doi: 10.4103/0253-7176.119477.

4. M. M. Shores et al., "Low Serum Testosterone and Mortality in Male Veterans," *Archives of Internal Medicine* 166 (2006): 1660–1665, doi: doi:10.1001/archinte.166.15.1660.
5. G. A. Laughlin et al., "Low Serum Testosterone and Mortality in Older Men," *Journal of Clinical Endocrinology and Metabolism* 93 (2008): 68–75, doi: 10.1210/jc.2007-1792.
6. When a man is being treated with testosterone replacement, the body senses that there's plenty of T now circulating, so it shuts down its own natural production of the hormone. A side effect is that it also shuts down production of sperm to some extent. Therefore, taking testosterone in any form can decrease fertility in men.
7. A. Morgantaler, "Testosterone and Prostate Cancer: What Are the Risks for Middle-Aged Men?," *Urologic Clinics of North America* 38 (2011): 119–124, doi: 10.1016/j.ucl.2011.02.002.
8. D. J. Jang et al., "Red Ginseng for Treating Erectile Dysfunction: A Systematic Review," *British Journal of Clinical Pharmacology* 66, no. 4 (2008): 444–450, doi: 10.1111/j.1365-2125.2008.03236.x.
9. B. C. Shin et al., "Maca (*L. meyenii*) for Improving Sexual Function: A Systematic Review," *BMC Complementary and Alternative Medicine* 10 (2010): 44, doi: 10.1186/1472-6882-10-44.

Resources

The Men's Health Network offers lots of great information about sexual health issues for men: www.MensHealthNetwork.org.

Men's Health Forum, a UK-based site, is full of great resources and has an active online support community: www. Menshealthforum.org/UK; another support site is www.Healthunlocked.com.

There are dozens of websites offering free advice on anabolic steroids for fat loss and muscle gain. Before following any of the advice you find online, ask a trusted medical professional. Info from the National Institutes of Health: https://www.drugabuse.gov/publications/drugfacts/anabolic-steroids.

Guidelines from the American Urological Association Guidelines on the use of testosterone: www.AUAnet.org/TestosteroneGuideline.

12

Optimal Brain Health

've said before that health is not the end in and of itself; rather, it is a tool, perhaps the most important tool we have, to help us achieve our goals. And optimal health is all about having that tool of health be the most effective it can be. When it's framed that way, you see that, as important as optimal health of the physical body is, brain health is especially essential to keeping us on track in life, as memory and staying sharp are vital.

There is naturally much concern among many men not only about truly devastating diseases such as Alzheimer's but also about the gradual decline of brain function as we age. Most physicians say they have little to offer patients in terms of prevention of age-related memory loss or cognitive power, but I would respectfully disagree—we are actually living at an exciting time in this regard. There is more and more research into ways to preserve brain function as we age that we can take advantage of and that will be presented in this chapter.

While most of the chapter will focus on the prevention of accelerated brain aging manifesting as loss of memory or cognitive abilities (ability to concentrate and process information), I want to start with the biggest elephant in the room regarding brain aging: dementia, especially Alzheimer's disease. Dementia is an overall term for many symptoms, such as difficulty with thinking, problem-solving, or language, that impact the ability to perform everyday activities and involve impaired reasoning and personality changes as well as memory loss. Most dementia is progressive, meaning symptoms gradually worsen as brain cells become damaged and die; however, there are some reversible dementia-like conditions caused by vitamin deficiencies, thyroid or other hormonal disorders, heavy metal buildup, infections, severe sleep disorders, or psychiatric conditions. This is why it is important for anyone with even early signs of dementia to have a full medical workup to make sure there are no such underlying conditions that need to be treated.

In terms of the less easily reversible dementia conditions, there are many causes, including Alzheimer's, vascular dementia (due to multiple small strokes), Parkinson's disease, and repeated head trauma, to name just a few. Alzheimer's disease (AD) is the most common, accounting for 70–90 percent of all dementias and affecting more than five million people in the United States, with half a million dying each year from it. AD is characterized by brain lesions (plaques) made up of a substance called beta-amyloid, as well as by a buildup of neurofibrillary tangles related to abnormalities in something called tau protein. It used to be thought that the damage in AD was caused only by these plaques and tangles, which blocked signaling as well as killing off neurons. Now, though, we understand that much of the damage is caused not only directly by these lesions but also by the inflammation triggered by the plaques. We have heard about the damage inflammation causes in other parts of the body—contributing to heart disease, for example—and it is no different in the brain. Furthermore, the inflammation from plaques in AD also interferes with the function of mitochondria (the parts of cells that make energy for the whole system to run) and neurotransmitters. Therefore, preventing the buildup of beta-amyloid or helping to clear it out, minimizing inflammation, promoting mitochondrial function, and correcting neurotransmitter imbalance are all key ways to help prevent AD or minimize its impact.[1]

ALZHEIMER'S DISEASE

- Alzheimer's disease is by far the most common cause of dementia.
- Alzheimer's can be prevented and ameliorated to some degree. Things that help:
  - Minimizing plaque buildup

- Clearing plaque that has developed
- Decreasing inflammation in the brain
- Protecting mitochondria in brain cells from damage
- Providing the brain with supportive nutrients
- Clearing toxic substances from the brain

Dr. Dale Bredesen writes about powerful ways to prevent and even reverse cognitive decline from AD in his book *The End of Alzheimer's*. His ReCODE (reversal of cognitive decline) aims to prevent the buildup of amyloid plaque, which he argues is triggered by the body's response to toxins—infections, toxic chemicals in food and the environment, metals, biotoxins, and the inflammatory response these provoke—as well as by a lack of supportive nutrients. He describes four different types of Alzheimer's, depending on whether it is a result of insufficient nutrients, high blood sugar, toxins, or high amounts of inflammation, all of which would be addressed somewhat differently.

The approach was initially described in an article published in 2016 in the journal *Aging*, describing the improvement in ten patients using his combined approach of medications, supplements, diet, and lifestyle interventions.[2] ReCODE involves addressing the multiple factors that lead to cognitive decline. Advanced lab tests identify the issues needing treatment.[3] The earlier treatment begins, whether with medications or the other elements of the ReCODE program, the greater the chance of completely reversing the cognitive changes.

Others, including Dr. Rudolph Tanzi, a neurologist at Harvard University and chair of the Genetics and Aging Research Unit at Massachusetts General Hospital, agree that the accumulation of plaques in AD may be an attempt by the brain to protect itself from a toxin or infection. Tanzi is working to understand the role of infections in triggering beta-amyloid plaque production, the development of neurofibrillary tangles to also develop, and inflammation.[4]

The approach I have learned from my training in functional and integrative medicine is also about treating the underlying causes of AD, and has served my patients well. Whether the patient's goal is to prevent cognitive decline or the patient is already experiencing memory or cognition issues, we look at the influences on brain health to see what needs to be improved. For anyone experiencing cognitive symptoms, such as memory

> **Box 12.1 Advanced Testing Related to Cognitive Decline**
>
> 1. Blood sugar testing (glucose, hemoglobin A1C, fasting insulin levels)
> 2. Inflammatory levels (C-reactive protein, ferritin, sed rate)
> 3. Autoimmune markers
> 4. Heavy metal levels
> 5. Genetic tests for ApoE, and other genetic tests related to detoxification processes
> 6. Food sensitivity testing, especially for gluten sensitivity
> 7. Leaky gut testing
> 8. Micronutrient levels

loss or difficulty processing information, Box 12.1 lists some of the tests I recommend considering, depending on your own risk factors. Many are not covered by insurance, so you may not need all of them, and you certainly don't need to do all of them at once. Try to find an integrative medicine practitioner who can guide you toward the tests that would be most relevant—not only to brain health but to other health conditions as well.

Dr. Bredesen's book and his ReCODE program show that this type of integrative medicine approach—testing for specific issues and then targeting an array of interventions based on the results—can be powerful in terms of preventing cognitive decline and even reversing it. This offers guidance and hope for those wanting to prevent AD and other types of dementia, especially those who are at high risk for AD, and for anyone already experiencing mild cognitive impairment.

The ApoE4 Gene

Of all the genetic tests that are available, the test for ApoE may be the most important. This is a gene on chromosome 19 that affects how fats are carried and dealt with in the body. As mentioned in Chapter 2, it affects risk for both heart disease and Alzheimer's disease. There are three versions of this gene: ApoE2, ApoE3, and ApoE4. The most common is ApoE3. If you are lucky enough to have the ApoE2 version, either from one or both parents (remember, you get two copies of each gene), you have lower than average risk for these diseases. But the ApoE4 version increases risk for both heart disease and AD. About 25 percent of Americans have one copy of ApoE4, which increases risk by about four times, while 2–3 percent have two copies, which increases risk more than tenfold. Also, age of onset is usually younger in people with the gene.

The test for this gene is widely available, but for a long time most people were not interested in knowing if they were at higher risk, because doctors told them there was nothing they could do to avoid dementia, and given that, knowing they had an increased chance of developing it would only cause anxiety and worry. But what if you knew that you *could* do something about it?

MATT: KNOWLEDGE IS POWER

Matt, a healthy forty-two-year-old with two young children, came to me for an optimal health assessment because he wanted to do anything he could to prevent health problems. For Matt, knowledge is power—and he wanted to know the exact state of his health as well as any potential problems that could be lurking around the corner for himself or that might have been passed down to his kids.

We performed genetic testing to determine any increased risk for heart disease, metabolic syndrome, diabetes, cancer, and Alzheimer's, among other conditions. When we got Matt's results, it turned out he had two copies of the ApoE4 gene. This wasn't a complete shock to Matt, as his mother had been diagnosed with AD in her early sixties.

Because of his mother's experience, Matt knew that there are a few medications used to minimize symptoms of AD, but they don't work for long or even all that well, and they have unpleasant side effects. So there was really no reasonable pharmaceutical solution for me to offer Matt when he had no symptoms. But I was able to recommend that we test for any issues that could contribute to the development of AD, using tests listed in Box 12.1. We found that he did have relatively high levels of inflammation and that some of his nutrient levels were low—nutrients that are important in detoxification. His ability to fight oxidative damage was also low.

We worked on getting Matt on an anti-inflammatory diet, added supplements to replenish the vitamins and minerals he needed, and put him on other supplements that help with detoxification. I recommended he eat more cruciferous vegetables, such as broccoli sprouts, that help boost the ability to fight oxidative damage. Step by step we worked on elements of his lifestyle that were not optimized for someone at the higher risk he was found to have (sleep, stress management, and exercise, for example). I feel confident this will help him avoid getting Alzheimer's at least until very old age, even with his genetic predispositions.

Remember, we are not victims of our genes. As the saying goes, genes load the gun, but we pull the trigger. I was able to give Matt tools he could use to prevent pulling that trigger. Seventy-five million Americans carry at least one copy of the ApoE4 gene, and I recommend you get tested for it. If you are positive, it may give you the incentive you need to pursue a similar program.

The program each man follows is individualized according to his own specific issues. MRI imaging using special software can be used to measure brain volume in the areas where brain-aging-associated cognitive decline is most often seen.[5] Following a program like ReCODE, and even doing aspects of such a program such as an eight-week mindfulness course, has been shown to actually regrow those parts of the brain.

I'd like to expand on some of the most generalizable elements of an optimal brain plan, as laid out in Box 12.2. Not everyone may need to balance hormones, reduce levels of heavy metals, or heal the gut, but some of these recommended approaches do apply to everyone and are applicable not only to preventing or reversing AD but also to maintaining optimal brain function in general. But first, a little bit about how it's even possible to impact how the brain functions with interventions like these.

Box 12.2 Preventing or Reversing Cognitive Decline

Work with your physician to determine what issues are contributing most to any cognitive impairment (toxins, infections, lack of nutrients or the right hormones, inflammation, high blood sugar), but in general, an approach might include:

- Spplements to support clearing of toxins and optimizing antioxidant power, maintain normal vitamin and mineral levels, and decrease inflammation and homocysteine
- Anti-inflammatory diet that eliminates gluten and sugar
- Good-quality sleep of seven to nine hours a night (make sure you don't have sleep apnea)
- Stress management daily, such as mindfulness meditation
- Brain training (see recommendations under Resources)
- Gut healing
- Hormonal balance
- Healthy mineral levels with low heavy metals
- Detoxification optimization, especially if genes point to issues with this
- Keeping blood sugar, weight, and blood pressure at normal levels

Neuroplasticity

When it comes to your brain, you actually *can* teach an old dog new tricks. Once thought to be immutable after early childhood, the brain actually has a remarkable ability to change and heal itself. Known as neuroplasticity, this ability to remodel itself depends at least in part on how our environment, behavior, and habits, and even our thoughts and feelings, impact the brain over the course of our lives.

In the 1970s, studies began to show the brain rewiring itself as the result of a person's experiences. At the University of California, San Francisco, Dr. Michael Merzenich found that the area of the brain usually responsible for processing input from a specific body part—say, the eyes, or an arm—developed different linkages or was assigned another function when a person was unable to use that body part. Subsequently, human trials and clinical experience have proven this ability to rewire the brain. For example, stroke or brain trauma patients can increase nerve stimulation to unaffected limbs through physical therapy and can retrain damaged limbs by recruiting healthy neurons to take over from the ones that stopped functioning. For example, for a right-handed person, loss of the ability to use the right hand would lead to rewiring of the brain to increase impulses to the part of the brain responsible for movement of the left hand.

A review of studies looking at the impact of physical activity on the brain showed that exercise improves brain function by causing changes in the brain itself.[6] People who exercised aerobically for a year had changes especially in the hippocampus and prefrontal cortex, the parts of the brain responsible for memory and for higher executive functions and moods. This means that exercise can decrease cognitive and psychiatric problems such as dementia and depression. Psychiatrist and researcher Dr. Norman Doidge wrote about neuroplasticity and the ways in which people can rewire their brains to increase their mental strength in his 2007 book, *The Brain That Changes Itself*, featuring case studies of patients who, without operations or medications, were able to reverse neurological decline and outlining the research that backs up their experiences. The science on neuroplasticity has only increased since his book was published.

I bring up neuroplasticity because it is through this process that lifestyle and diet can actually help to rewire the brain in ways that both prevent and reverse dementia and the negative impacts of aging on the brain. It's also pertinent to the various types of Alzheimer's Bredesen mentions, because neuroplasticity can work both ways—the brain can be rewired in ways that are beneficial, but outside influences such as toxins, infections, and stress can also rewire our brains in ways that affect us negatively. For example, the more reactive we are, the more reactive we will continue to be, because we are reinforcing pathways that lead from feeling stressed to being easily emotionally triggered. Some of our most stubborn habits and unhealthy behaviors—and therefore some of our disorders—are products of our neuroplasticity. But let's look at things you can do to make beneficial changes in the brain.

Diet

As was mentioned, a large contributor to dementia is inflammation in the brain. So if you are serious about preventing or reversing cognitive decline or dementia, then you must minimize inflammation in as many ways as possible. An unhealthy diet is arguably the most common cause of inflammation in the body and brain (assuming there are no other causes such as toxins, heavy metals, or infections). The anti-inflammatory diet is discussed at length in Chapter 3, so I won't repeat that information here. But be aware that the most inflammatory parts of your diet are gluten and sugar, so if you are looking to boost cognition, be mindful of how much gluten and sugar you consume.

Many sources suggest that a gluten-free diet is hugely important in optimizing brainpower, especially Dr. David Perlmutter, a leading integrative neurologist and author of the book *Grain Brain.* Both Drs. Bredesen and Perlmutter cite evidence of the negative impact of gluten and sugar on the brain. In fact, Perlmutter and others consider AD to be "type 3 diabetes" (type 1 is insulin-dependent diabetes and type 2 is related to insulin resistance). A combination of insulin resistance and insulin deficiency in the brain has been shown to increase the inflammation that causes and worsens the cognitive decline seen in dementia. Furthermore, insulin resistance has other effects that contribute directly to cognitive impairment.

In addition to the recommendation to maintain an anti-inflammatory diet, avoid gluten, and minimize sugar as much as possible, there is some evidence for other specific diets for particular neurologic conditions that affect the brain. Dr. Terry Wahls is a physician who was diagnosed with multiple sclerosis (MS), leading her to investigate diets that would ultimately help her reverse the course of her disease. She has spoken about her approach in a compelling TED talk and has written about it in her book

The Wahls Protocol. Her work has not generated the amount of research done by Perlmutter or Bredesen, but for MS specifically it is worth looking at her protocol, which utilizes a version of the paleo diet.[7]

In terms of diets that might be useful for Alzheimer's prevention, the ketogenic diet has the greatest number of proponents. The ketogenic diet has been successful in children with epilepsy, and there is evidence that it can be useful for dementia prevention and treatment. This is not absolutely proven yet, but because glucose metabolism is severely impaired in many people with Alzheimer's (remember that AD is considered by many to be a form of diabetes), a diet extremely low in carbohydrates, such as the ketogenic diet, may be helpful. I am not necessarily advocating it, as the jury is still out in terms of long-term impact, but I would be remiss in not mentioning it, as it is an area of intense study.[8]

What about fasting? It is true that restricting calories in general helps with longevity. This will be discussed in Chapter 14, on optimal aging. Researchers have studied some variations on fasting, such as intermittent fasting (restricting eating to a limited period of time, such as eight or nine hours within a twenty-four-hour period). It is thought that the mechanism through which caloric restriction decreases cellular aging is its impact on sirtuin function. Sirtuins are a family of molecules that influence genes in ways that affect aging, especially cellular aging, throughout the body and brain. Activating sirtuins through caloric restriction can decrease cellular aging. I bring this up because I anticipate more research and discussion in the near future about the role of diet and supplements in activating this very important pathway.

Stress Management

Stress is toxic to the brain. Chronic stress keeps cortisol elevated, and cortisol has been shown to kill off brain cells when it stays high. Research shows that stress especially decreases normal function in the prefrontal cortex, the part of the brain responsible for rational decision-making and appropriate responses to situations. Do you notice how when you get angry your ability to think clearly and respond in a rational way flies out the window—instead of responding in a measured manner, you react like an animal? The prefrontal cortex is actually what differentiates us from animals, so when we allow ourselves to get so triggered that we shut off this executive function rooted in the prefrontal cortex, we lose the ability to respond appropriately, and instead simply react unconsciously.

But there are ways to decrease the toxic effect of stress by reclaiming the power to control our own thoughts instead of allowing our thoughts to control us. One of the most powerful ways is through mindfulness meditation, as discussed in Chapter 6. Programs such as mindfulness-based stress reduction have been proven to decrease the impact of stress on the brain and body by eliciting the relaxation response, which decreases the amount of cortisol and helps to protect the brain.

A regular stress management program, which may include yoga, breath work, journaling, or tai chi, is indicated for prevention of age-related cognitive decline and reversal of early age-related changes. In fact, it has been shown that regular meditation can improve attention span and can help you to remain attentive and focused well into old age.[9] When stress is reduced, your neuroplasticity increases.

Physical Activity

Evidence is mounting that physical exercise is good for the brain as well as the body—and it's from more than the increase in endorphins that comes from intense cardio (often called runner's high). Aerobic exercise actually slows the loss of gray matter, the type of cells that make up the cerebral cortex (the outer layer of brain), responsible for information processing. Gray matter atrophies as you age, so exercising helps keep that part of the brain alive and engaged. In fact, higher gray matter volume is correlated with intelligence and skill at certain activities, depending on the location in the brain. For example, London taxi drivers showed increased volume in the area of the brain known for spatial navigation, with the increase in size correlating with years of driving. You're probably not a London taxi driver, but this example show that more volume in brain cortex means generally better functioning, and physical exercise increases brain volume.

It has also been shown that anaerobic exercise, such as resistance or strength training, stimulates the creation of new brain cells in the hippocampus, the part of the brain responsible for memory and learning. Furthermore, we know that stress can kill off brain cells in this same region. So when you consider that exercise helps relieve stress as well, you see how important exercise is to the brain.

There are other ways in which exercise is neuroprotective, meaning it builds up our ability to defend ourselves against neurological decline. Exercise causes levels of a substance called brain-derived neurotrophic factor (BDNF) to increase. BDNF has been called "Miracle-Gro for the brain" by Harvard psychiatrist John J. Ratey, MD, in his book *Spark: The Revolutionary New Science of Exercise and the Brain* because it helps nerve cells transmit information better. In fact, low levels of BDNF are associated with depression, so increasing BDNF through exercise can be a natural antidepressant—much more permanent than that surge of endorphins.

One more way that exercise helps the brain is by preventing brain damage from stroke. Many studies attest to the benefit of cardiovascular exercise in preventing or minimizing atherosclerosis, the process by which arteries get clogged with plaque. Strokes occur when such plaque-ridden arteries interfere with blood flow to the brain. One recent study showed that men engaging in intense physical activity had less than half the risk of stroke as those who did not engage in such activities. Furthermore, for those who did have a stroke, the ones who had been exercising before the stroke recovered more fully and faster than those who were not physically active. So exercise was like an insurance policy that both protected people against stroke and helped them get better even if they did have one.

Brainpower: Use It or Lose It

There is evidence that we may prevent symptoms of dementia and brain aging by remaining socially engaged and intellectually curious throughout our lives. Rudy Tanzi, PhD, and Deepak Chopra, MD, explored the power of our brains in their book *Super Brain*. The brain needs healthy food as nourishment and avoidance of toxins and stress, but also mental challenges. This is not mere supposition, but actually has been proven over and over again in studies showing that remaining engaged in mental activity and maintaining strong social connections help to preserve brain function.

Supplements

Once the stuff of science fiction, pills to make us smarter may now be a reality. Neurotropics are compounds that enhance cognitive functions like memory, motivation, and creativity. Prescription "smart drugs" like Adderall (amphetamine combination) and Provigil (modafinil) are well known and used everywhere from college campuses to Silicon Valley, even though they are meant for specific conditions such as attention deficit disorder. It is dangerous to use these without a prescription, for inappropriate indications, and without the guidance of a medical professional. But natural compounds can also act as brain enhancers. These are generally called nootropics—amino acids, minerals, or other nutrients that don't have the side effects or toxicity of general neurotropics and are more neuroprotective. One example of a nootropic is caffeine. You probably already use caffeine to help keep you sharp—most of us aren't functional before that first cup of coffee every morning. Caffeine is considered a nootropic, in that it does improve mental sharpness and even learning ability. Other supplements that act as nootropics include:

- L-theanine, a compound found in black and green tea, on its own can help you relax without making you tired, helping to bring on a state of relaxed alertness. When paired with caffeine, it works synergistically to increase memory and improve reaction time.[10]
- Bacopa, an herb used in Ayurvedic medicine, has been shown to enhance attention and mood in older people as well as improve memory in healthy adults.
- Lion's mane, a medicinal mushroom used in Chinese medicine, is one of the more powerful nootropics, enhancing nerve growth factor and helping with memory and focus.
- Piracetam, a derivative of the neurotransmitter GABA, improves neuroplasticity and has neuroprotective effects. Together with oxiracetam, it helps with focus and concentration.
- Oxiracetam, similar in function to piracetam, helps especially to improve memory and is considered the strongest substance in the racetam family.
- Noopept is similar to piracetam, but more potent.
- Pterostilbene, found naturally in blueberries, is an antioxidant similar to resveratrol (found in red wine) but more bioavailable. It is neuroprotective and activates sirtuin 1, a molecule linked to longevity.
- NAD$^+$ (nicotinamide riboside) becomes depleted with age, causing a decline in activity of sirtuins. Taking NAD is said to activate sirtuins. [11]

There are other supplements that are not necessarily nootropics per se but can help prevent cognitive decline. For example, fish oil contains the omega-3 fatty acids DHA and EPA, which are critical for neurological development and function. Many studies have looked at the ability of omega-3s to mitigate age-related deterioration of the brain, with interesting results. In one animal study, DHA and EPA supplementation reversed changes related to aging and maintained learning memory performance. Another study of older adults found that people who took a DHA supplement for six months showed improvements in learning and memory. I generally recommend a dose of 2,000 mg of combined EPA and DHA daily.

L-carnitine is an often-depleted enzyme that plays an important role in converting food into energy. Supplementing with this enzyme (in the form of acetyl-L-carnitine) may help slow down cognitive decline associated with aging. In fact, a meta-analysis of studies looking at supplementation with acetyl-L-carnitine for periods ranging from three to twelve months showed beneficial effects for people with mild cognitive impairment as well as those with early Alzheimer's disease. Generally 1,000 mg a day is an adequate dose, but it should be of the acetyl-L-carnitine form.

The Bottom Line

Through a modern understanding of neuroplasticity and the ways that we can influence brain health, we are actually more in control of brain aging than was ever thought possible. Our diet, our activity, habits of mental and social engagement, efforts at managing stress, and our ability to boost energy production, detoxify, and minimize inflammation through supplementation all make huge a difference in how we use the amazing organ that is responsible for our creativity, memory, sense perceptions, and capacity for abstract thought. Even if you already are experiencing memory loss, it is not too late to reverse any decline in brain function.

Questions to Ask Your Doctor

First of all, let me say that I don't recommend simply chalking up any change in memory, concentration, or processing of information to "old age." You should discuss any such changes with your doctor. As this chapter discusses, there may be reversible issues that can make a big difference in brain function. With that in mind, if you are noticing a decline in cognitive function, consider asking your doctor these questions.

1. What tests do you recommend for objectively assessing and keeping track of my brain function? (I use one by Cambridge Brain Sciences in my practice.)
2. Would you recommend I have an MRI scan with quantification of the parts of my brain responsible for memory? (I use one called NeuroQuant.)
3. Are there any neurological side effects from current medications I am taking that could affect brain health?

4. Should I be taking any supplements to help my brain function better? (Ask about any supplements you are considering, including the ones mentioned in this chapter.)
5. Should I be tested for heavy metals, hormones, or inflammation? (If you are having symptoms, the answer may be yes.)
6. Should I see a specialist? (If you have high risk based on genes or have been diagnosed with Alzheimer's, ask about referrals to specialists who are familiar with newer approaches such as Dr. Bredesen's ReCODE program.)

Notes

1. More on the cause, or pathophysiology, of Alzheimer's Disease can be found on the video "Alzheimer's Disease—Plaques, Tangles, Causes, Symptoms and Pathology," posted by Osmosis, March 22, 2016, : https://www.youtube.com/watch?v=v5gdH_Hydes.
2. D. E. Bredesen et al., "Reversal of Cognitive Decline in Alzheimer's Disease," *Aging* 8, no. 6 (2016): 1–9, doi: 10.18632/aging.100981.
3. Lab tests that can be useful in directing a program aimed at reversing cognitive decline should be individualized, but might include:

Homocysteine
B vitamin and vitamin E levels
Fasting glucose and insulin levels
CRP
Ratio of omega-6 to omega-3
Albumin-to-globulin ratio
IL-6 and TNF-alpha
Vitamin D_3 level
Full hormone panel
Copper and zinc
RBC magnesium
Selenium
Glutathione
Heavy metal panel
Lipid panel
Food sensitivities
Neuropsychiatric testing
Gut and blood-brain barrier permeability

These may not all be covered by traditional medical insurance or available to be ordered by every physician. Some of these tests are more often ordered by an integrative medicine physician.

4. Interesting article about Tanzi's work and the probability of infections being part of the cause of AD: Alvin Powell, "Probe of Alzheimer's Follows Path of Infection," *Harvard Gazette*, May 2017, https://news.harvard.edu/gazette/story/2017/05/devastating-chain-of-events-found-in-alzheimers-path.

5. MRI software such as NeuroQuant enables a radiologist and neurologist to quantify parts of the brain being affected by disease, such as the volume of the hippocampus, which is one of the most important parts of the brain involved in memory. Shrinkage of the hippocampus directly correlates with memory loss.

6. K. I. Erickson, A. G. Gildengers, and M. A. Butters, "Physical Activity and Brain Plasticity in Late Adulthood," *Dialogues in Clinical Neuroscience* 15, no. 1 (2013): 99–108.

7. There are links to articles on the paleo diet on the site https://terrywahls.com. Keep in mind that she is finding articles that support her own ideas about paleo, specifically for MS.

8. A ketogenic diet is a diet so low in carbohydrates that the body switches to using fat as a source of fuel instead of the normal use of carbs. In this diet, all sweeteners, starchy carbohydrates, and grains are removed, and minimal fruit is eaten; the emphasis is on fats from clean animal sources (beef and milk from grass-fed hormone-free cows, organic chicken and eggs, wild fish), nuts and seeds, and MCT oil (no hydrogenated oils or oils high in omega-6-fatty acids, such as canola, corn, sunflower, safflower, or soy oils).

9. A. P. Zanesco et al., "Cognitive Aging and Long-Term Maintenance of Attentional Improvements Following Meditation Training," *Journal of Cognitive Enhancement* 2, no. 3 (2018): 259–275, doi: 10.1007/s41465-018-0068-1.

10. D. A. Camfield et al., "Acute Effects of Tea Constituents L-theanine, Caffeine, and Epigallocatechin Gallate on Cognitive Function and Mood: A Systematic Review and Meta-Analysis," *Nutrition Reviews* 72, no.8 (2014): 507–522, doi: 10.1111/nure.12120.

11. There is a combination of nootropics in a formula developed by scientists at UCLA and available to the general public called TruBrain. The science behind this formula is impressive but still preliminary. Initial research has shown that it improved brain wave activity, enhanced verbal fluency, and improved memory.

Resources

Cambridge Brain Sciences (https://www.cambridgebrainsciences.com/
science/tests) offers a neurocognitive test battery that can provide
objective measures of any deficiencies in concentration, reasoning,
short-term memory, or verbal ability. These tests must be administered
by a medical provider. They can be used to track progress as you
implement recommendations discussed in this chapter.

Info on a ketogenic diet is available from Dr. David Perlmutter's website,
https://www.drperlmutter.com/ketogenic-diet-benefits.

There is much information about the effects of fasting on aging in the book
The Longevity Diet, by Victor Longo (New York: Avery, 2018).

Activities that can help to keep memory and cognition sharp:

- Using memory software or apps for brain training, like Lumosity, www.
  lumosity.com.
- Doing crossword puzzles
- Playing bridge
- Solving Rubik's cube
- Reading
- Taking a class
- Exercising
- Learning a foreign language

13

Optimal Fitness

Exercise is good for you. It's one of the most important of our eight levers for optimal health, as I discuss in Chapter 5. You really don't need to look any further than number one on the list of benefits of exercise in Box 5.1: prevention of premature death. People who are very active (at least three hours per week of vigorous activity, such as sports or high-intensity gardening tasks such as digging or raking) have a lower risk of dying early than those who are active for less than thirty minutes a week. Many studies have shown this; one large study showed that the most active men added four years to their life compared to inactive men. And it's never too late to start: this same study showed that going from sedentary to active between ages fifty and sixty adds 1.6 years to life expectancy. Even those who start exercising in their sixties get benefits, such as a 32 percent lower risk of developing mild cognitive impairment.[1] My final pitch for the benefit of exercise relates to sex: a review in the *Journal of Andrology* looking at multiple studies found that physical activity reduces erectile dysfunction.[2]

But this chapter focuses more on exercise as a means to achieve fitness goals and as a powerful tool to make sure optimal health is enabling you to achieve whatever goals you have. As a reminder, I recommend a mix of physical activity to gain all of the benefits possible:

- Cardiovascular exercise, such as biking, running, using an elliptical machine, or anything that gets your heart rate up for the duration of your exercise. Intervals (alternating faster-paced activity with a slower pace) are best for weight loss and overall fitness.
- Core exercises—sit-ups, planks, yoga, and Pilates—strengthen your abdominal muscles and lower back, which helps to prevent low back pain.
- Resistance training—weightlifting or bodyweight exercises such as pull-ups, push-ups, or yoga—helps increase bone strength and muscle mass, which can increase basal metabolic rate (helping you to burn more calories throughout the day). It also boosts testosterone levels, which in turn makes it easier to gain more muscle mass.
- Flexibility—stretching and yoga help to prevent injury.

You may think you couldn't fit all these in your exercise regimen, but there are ways to kill two birds with one stone. For example, both yoga and tai chi can provide cardio, core, and flexibility work, and many yoga poses bring in bodyweight resistance as well.

If you're wondering what the least amount of exercise is you can do and still get some health benefits, there's some good news. Recent studies show that short but very intense bursts of cardiovascular exercise can be as beneficial as longer bouts of less intense activity. In fact, one study showed that ten minutes of high-intensity interval training proved to be as successful at improving health and fitness as forty-five minutes of moderate exercise. Scientists at McMaster University in Hamilton, Ontario, divided young men into two groups. One group exercised for forty-five minutes at 75 percent of maximum heart rate, and the other did an interval workout, pedaling as hard as they could for twenty seconds, followed by two minutes of easy pedaling, repeated three times, for a total of only ten minutes, including warm-up and cool-down. After twelve weeks, the two groups of exercisers had nearly identical gains. In both groups, endurance had increased by nearly 20 percent, insulin resistance had improved, and there were significant increases in muscle function related to energy production and oxygen consumption. I can't say if short bursts like that will provide all the long-term effects of exercise I've described, but it does mean that even if you think you have no time to exercise, finding merely ten minutes a day a few times a week for a high-intensity workout can make a big difference in your fitness.[3]

MIKE: HITTING HIS GOAL

Mike, whom we talked about in Chapter 1, wanted to coach his kid's soccer team, but he was out of shape and overweight, so he couldn't keep up with the kids enough to help coach. He needed to have sufficient stamina to run up and down the field during practice. Mike had a hard time getting the motivation to go the gym, and when there, he wasn't sure what to do in order to make the best use of his time and effort. He didn't have the money for a personal trainer. I suggested he try a group class, like CrossFit, boot camp, or Orangetheory. He tried it but felt like he wasn't ready for these. Fortunately, most trainers will work with small groups of people at one time, which makes the price much more reasonable for each person. I have a trainer who will put four people together to work out as a group for an hour or so. For Mike, that did the trick. He has been working out once or twice a week with the group, learning what to do and being pushed much harder than he would push himself. After only six months he was able to be an assistant coach for his son's soccer team.

Supplements and Exercising

What about supplements to gain more benefits from exercise in terms of weight loss, muscle development, general toning, and improving strength, speed, or overall performance?

Creatine. Naturally produced in the human body, creatine is taken up preferentially by muscle cells, where it is used for production of ATP, a substance that provides energy to cells. Creatine does seem to increase the size of muscle cells; theoretically this increases muscle strength, but that hasn't been proven. Extensive research has shown that supplementation at the amounts generally recommended for muscle strength does not cause adverse side effects, Still, those with kidney disease or at risk for kidney disease are generally advised against using it.

Taurine. An amino acid naturally found in the body, taurine has been touted as an energy booster. While small studies have shown some improvement in VO_{2max} (one indicator of fitness) after daily use of taurine as a supplement, there have not been consistent findings of benefit from its use.

Branched-chain amino acids. Branched-chain amino acids (BCAAs), which include leucine, isoleucine, and valine, have similarly been used to improve athletic performance. Supplemental intake of these amino acids is purported to decrease exercise-induced muscle damage, increase muscle recovery, and help to build lean muscle mass in response to strength training. There is some evidence that supplemental BCAAs do have anabolic effects, meaning they may help to build muscle. BCAAs seem to be a safe supplement to take, with no serious adverse side effects.

DHEA. A natural androgenic hormone produced in the adrenal glands, DHEA has been recommended in doses ranging from 10 to 100 mg a day for anabolic and antiaging effects. While DHEA may improve lean muscle mass due to its androgenic effects, there is no evidence that it improves athletic performance.

Acetyl-L-carnitine. Carnitine is a frequently depleted enzyme that plays a critical role in the Krebs cycle, which powers everything in your body by converting food into energy. Research suggests supplementing with acetyl-L-carnitine can have a beneficial effect on athletic training, competition, and recovery. In one study looking at the effects of acute carnitine loading on professional athletes, those who were given the supplement before performing a running test showed increased speed and decreased heart rate compared to a placebo group.[4] Taking 1,000 mg of acetyl-L-carnitine every day can improve your ability to make energy in your cells, translating to energy for your workouts.

Ginseng. As discussed in Chapter 4, on supplements, there are several types of ginseng. The type most proven to help with athletic performance and fitness is *Panax ginseng* (also known as Asian or Korean ginseng). It is one of the most thoroughly studied herbs for athletic performance. Taking about 1,000 mg a day can help to enhance gains in muscle strength from working out and to decrease exercise-induced fatigue, thereby increasing stamina. Another aspect of exercise that ginseng helps is muscle recovery: ginseng helps the body repair oxidative damage to muscles after an intense workout.

Steroids

What about anabolic steroids? These include forms of testosterone that help muscles to get bigger in response to exercise. They generally need to be self-injected on a weekly basis and have to be taken along with other medications or supplements to minimize side effects such as testicular shrinkage and breast enlargement. I don't recommend their use because of potential adverse effects on the heart, including high blood pressure, heart attack, and stroke. Neurological side effects include anxiety, rage, depression, psychosis, and even suicidality. It is disheartening to hear that some teens are abusing these substances—surveys have shown that 5 percent or more of high school athletes illegally use anabolic steroids. This is particularly worrisome for this age group, because steroids heavily impact sexual function and development. For all ages, anabolic steroids affect testosterone production and can cause testicular atrophy and infertility. In addition to the all the side effects mentioned earlier, some guys who use them will develop acne or experience hair loss.[5]

Sports Injuries and Treatment

Increased physical activity can mean increased risk of injuries, so it's important to be aware of injuries related to exercise including overuse syndromes. Forty to 50 percent of runners, for example, suffer a running-related injury in any given year. It is important to listen to your body and to *not* buy in to the "no pain, no gain" philosophy. If you have pain, pull back from what you are doing and seek the help of a physical therapist, chiropractor, or podiatrist to help identify the problem. It may have to do with your anatomy or your exercise form.

Tendinitis and Tendinopathy

Some specific sports-related injuries that can be related to overuse injuries include tendinitis and tendinopathy. Tendinitis is usually related to an acute injury, such as trying to do a biceps curl with an extra-heavy weight; damage to the tendons results in inflammation and pain. Treatment is rest and anti-inflammatory medications or supplements such as turmeric or quercetin.

Tendinopathy is more common in middle-aged or elderly men engaging in physical activity and is usually related to overuse or repetitive strain on a tendon, such as embarking on an exercise program too aggressively, without building up slowly as the body gets stronger and stronger. In overuse tendinopathy, there is no traumatic damage and inflammation in the tendons, as there is with tendinitis. If you were to look at the affected tendon under a microscope, you wouldn't see inflammatory cells, as you do with tendinitis. You would see general disorganized cells with scar tissue, a problem called tendinosis. An anti-inflammatory approach doesn't work for these conditions.

ZACH: A CASE OF SHOULDER TENDINOPATHY

Zach came in complaining of left shoulder pain. When I examined him, he didn't have any swelling or warmth in the joint, but he couldn't lift his arm higher than his shoulder. He didn't remember any sudden "pop" or trauma, no sudden hard throwing or fall. The pain just came on over time. It was worst in the morning and radiated down his arm. Zach did sleep on his left side a lot, and it hurt when he lay on it. He played tennis regularly and had been working on his serves more recently. An MRI didn't show any tear, but he did have thickening of the tendons of one of the main muscles of the rotator cuff (the supraspinatus).

With a combination of acupuncture and physical therapy along with exercises at home (including "wall-walking," in which he had to gradually move his hand up a wall to extend his range of movement), he was much better after six weeks. He was able to avoid any steroid injections or even having to take anti-inflammatories, which might have helped a little but wouldn't have cured the problem.

Patients with tendinopathy complain of pain with activities that cause tendon loading, or the mechanical force that's applied to tendons when we move our muscles and joints. Joint stiffness and muscle weakness may occur. Common physical findings of tendinopathy include tenderness and thickening over the affected segment of the tendon. With time, the degenerated and weakened state of the tendon can lead to tendon rupture or tear. Acupuncture and manual therapies aimed at breaking up scar tissue and promoting blood flow into affected areas can be helpful with all tendinopathies. Let's take a look at some specific tendinopathies with their corresponding treatments.

Achilles Tendinopathy

Achilles tendinopathy is characterized by chronic heel pain and swelling. Pain is aggravated by tendon-loading activities, such as walking and running, and by external pressure caused by the back of the shoe. Common causes include overtraining, exercising on uneven surfaces, poor flexibility of the gastrocnemius (one of the calf muscles), overpronation of the foot, inappropriate footwear, and taking fluoroquinolone antibiotics (such as Cipro [ciprofloxacin] or Levaquin [levofloxacin]). Treatment includes avoidance of high-impact physical activity, heel lifts (inserts in shoes), and open-back shoes to reduce stress on the tendon. Eccentric training, characterized by stretching the tendon while under tension, has been shown to be beneficial. Corticosteroid injections are not recommended, as they may increase the risk of tendon rupture.

Rotator Cuff Tendinopathy

The rotator cuff muscles are important for shoulder movements and for stabilizing the shoulder joint. They consist of the four muscles that surround the shoulder joint: the supraspinatus, infraspinatus, teres minor, and subscapularis.

Risks for rotator cuff tendinopathy include repetitive overhead activity, such as in tennis, golf, and swimming, especially in men over fifty with some arthritis of the shoulder joint itself. It can be caused by microtrauma to the tendon or by bone spurs (osteophytes). Patients commonly report shoulder pain with overhead activity or while lying on the affected shoulder at night.

Treatment includes rest and avoidance of overhead activities. Physical therapy that focuses on range of motion and strengthening the rotator cuff muscles can be beneficial. Acupuncture can help, and recently injections with platelet-rich plasma (PRP) has been shown to be effective.[6] Surgical repair may be an option in severe situations.

Patellar Tendinopathy

Patients with patellar tendinopathy, commonly referred to as "jumper's knee," complain of pain in the front of the knee, especially when walking down stairs, running, or prolonged sitting.

Treatment includes avoidance of the activities that cause pain. No role has been found for braces or steroid injections, but PRP may be helpful here. Surgery is very rarely indicated.

Elbow Tendinopathy

A common tendinopathy, lateral elbow epicondylitis, is also known as tennis elbow. In this condition, there is pain in the forearm along the thumb side caused by damage to the tendons that bend the wrist away and back from the arm.

Treatment includes physical therapy and avoiding activities that require repetitive wrist flexion. Instruction on proper stroke mechanics and appropriate racket type can be beneficial to tennis players before returning to play. A forearm brace may help as well. Steroid injections may provide short-term relief of pain but do not prevent recurrence and may lead to worse long-term outcomes. A number of other potential therapies, including PRP and even Botox (botulinum toxin) injections, may be helpful.

Plantar Fasciitis

Plantar fasciitis is one of the most common causes of foot pain, especially in runners. It arises as a result of repetitive microtrauma to the plantar fascia, the connective tissue that lines the bottom of the feet, from excessive mechanical stress. With plantar fasciitis, people complain of pain in the heel or arch of the foot, typically worse the first time you put weight on it after getting up in the morning or after sitting for a long time. The pain gets better as the foot loosens up. If you have flat feet or high arches, or if you run a lot on hard surfaces without proper cushioning, you have a higher risk for this problem.

Treatment includes rest, shoe inserts to provide arch and heel support, and plantar fascia stretching. Icing may provide some pain relief—I often recommend patients keep a small plastic water bottle in the freezer and roll the ice-filled bottle against the bottom of their feet first thing in the morning. Also, it helps to avoid going barefoot or wearing flat shoes if you suffer from plantar fasciitis.

Monitoring Your Fitness

This section touches on some ways to monitor your level of fitness. With the popularity of wearable devices that monitor heart rate and many other measures, you may not be sure what to do with all the data you can now track regarding your own exercise and fitness. I do think it can be motivating to use a wearable device connected to an app to track your progress. I especially like apps where you can compete against others doing a similar workout or against yourself doing the same workout at different points in time. Strava is a great social competition app that allows you to do that, especially if you are a cyclist.

If you use wearables, the following are a few metrics that can be useful to track on your way to becoming more fit.

Resting Heart Rate (RHR)

Your heart rate in beats per minute (bpm), checked first thing in the morning before getting out of bed, can be a good indicator of overall physical fitness. Among nonathletes, it has been shown that a higher resting heart rate (at the higher end of the normal zone, which runs from 60 to 100 bpm) is linked with worse physical fitness and even a higher risk of premature death. A study published in the journal *Heart* in 2013 showed that a resting heart rate between 80 and 90 was associated with double the risk of death of those with lower resting heart rates, and those with an RHR between 90 and 100 had three times the risk of death.[7] But a heart rate that is consistently very low, especially in a nonathlete, could be a sign of an electrical problem with the heart, so that needs to be checked out.

What about for athletes? While the normal rate for resting heart rate is 60–100 bpm, it can be in the 40s or 50s in well-conditioned athletes. This lower rate indicates a more efficient heart—pumping more blood per beat, therefore requiring fewer beats per minute to get the needed amount of blood (and oxygen) circulating. While training can decrease RHR and increase efficiency, overtraining can cause fatigue, decreased efficiency, and a higher RHR. But once RHR is down in this low range, it hasn't been absolutely proven whether further decreases are truly meaningful in terms of overall cardiac fitness. So RHR is a meaningful indicator of fitness more for the amateur than for the elite runner or triathlete. For this latter group, VO_{2max} may be a more sensitive indicator of fitness.

Key MEASURES OF FITNESS

It's great to follow a measure of your fitness over time to gauge your improvement.

Recommended measures include:

Resting heart rate
VO_{2max}
Heart rate variability
Waist circumference

VO_{2max}

The best metric of aerobic fitness, VO_{2max} measures the maximum rate at which you can utilize the oxygen that you breathe in for fueling your muscles. The more you train, the more efficient you get at utilizing oxygen and therefore working your muscles maximally. When muscles run out of oxygen, they produce lactate—causing that burn you feel when you have reached your capacity. In order to go faster or be stronger, you need to increase how hard your muscles can work, and to do that, they need to be able to utilize oxygen more and more efficiently over time. Basically, VO_{2max} is your maximal aerobic capacity; the higher it is, the harder you can go. Elite athletes might have a VO_{2max} of over 80 mL/kg/min, while the fit amateur may be in the 50s; a higher-end amateur might be in the mid-60s. The weekend warrior is more around 40–50.

Even the American Heart Association said in 2017 that a measure of cardiorespiratory fitness like VO_{2max} should be considered a vital sign by doctors because low cardiorespiratory fitness is associated with higher risk for heart disease, dementia, diabetes, and even depression.[8]

It used to be very complicated to accurately measure VO_{2max}, requiring someone to run on a treadmill while hooked up to a mask with a hose attached to a computer, but now newer wearable devices can give you a pretty good indicator of your VO_{2max}. I love being able to see my VO_{2max} on a regular basis. It gives me the most accurate sense I've ever had of my true aerobic fitness.

Heart Rate Variability (HRV)

HRV is a proven measure of stress. The normal, healthy heart has some natural variability in the amount of time between beats. When you are stressed and the fight-or-flight reflex of your autonomic nervous system is kicking into high gear, the interval between heartbeats evens out to an unnatural degree, exhibiting minimal variability. This is a sign of an overall increased state of stress and decreased state of relaxation. So HRV can give you insight into how stressed your body is, even when you might not be feeling the rise in stress (because guys are notoriously bad at being in touch with their bodies and what's going on physiologically). Professional athletes are using HRV as a measure of stress to help determine how intensive a workout should be. Viewing HRV in real time helps you see the impact of drinking alcohol (which can lower HRV) or meditating (which has been proven to increase HRV), for example. Studies have even shown that low HRV increases risk of death after a heart attack.

One of the leaders in this is HeartMath, a nonprofit that sells sensors and has great information and studies on its website about the correlation between higher HRV and improved motor coordination and reaction times, clearer decision-making, and better performance in general. People who have higher HRV have greater resilience to stress. HRV can be improved with diet (green tea helps), yoga, meditation, exercise, and better sleep.

There are apps (like HeartMath's InnerBalance app or Elite HRV) that can be used to measure HRV using a chest strap or ear clip (the most accurate), and others that use a smartphone's camera. There are also wearable devices like Whoop (being used by Major League Baseball) and the Oura ring that can measure HRV accurately.

Waist Circumference

I recommend to my patients that they measure their waist circumference over time instead of their weight. If you are working out and your muscle mass increases, your weight won't reflect your loss of fat, because the increased muscle weighs more than the lost fat. Measure your waist with a tape measure at the level of your belly button midway between the in-breath and the out-breath. That will be a better marker of your progress.

The Bottom Line

This aim of this chapter is to give you a sense of the importance of exercise for your overall physical, mental, and even sexual health. Go ahead and try a ten-minute interval workout along with a couple of supplements. If you are new to exercise, the best way to cement a new healthy habit is to make a commitment for a few weeks, so I encourage you to find a chunk of time that works for you and commit! You may want to start with a baseline

EVEN IF YOU HATE THE GYM, YOU CAN EXERCISE

Maybe the gym is not for you. There are many ways to get the recommended physical activity for optimal health without stepping foot in a gym. Here are a few suggestions:

1. Swimming is excellent exercise, and most towns have a community pool.
2. Consider a dance class, especially one like Zumba or salsa, which will definitely get you breaking a sweat.
3. Try an at-home program that uses minimal equipment. There are many available online (see the Resources section).
4. If you have an active dog, go for a brisk walk or light jog with your canine friend.
5. If you live close to any hiking trails, even urban ones, take advantage of that. Walking uphill is like running on a flat surface—doing hills, like you'd find on a hike, can get your heart rate up there and get you conditioned just as easily as running.
6. If you have knee issues, a rower is a great piece of equipment to invest in for home use.

measure of your weight, waist circumference, and resting heart rate. Track them over time and see your health improve.

Questions to Ask Your Doctor

1. Am I doing this exercise right?
    (If you have any musculoskeletal pain as a result of exercise, seek help from a chiropractor, physical therapist, or yoga therapist, or ask your doctor about it. Many times you can minimize risk of injury just by doing an exercise a little differently.)
2. Is this exercise plan safe for me?
    (If you have any chronic medical problems, ask your doctor about your exercise plan. The doctor may have suggestions about how to gradually increase your fitness without risking your health in any way.)
3   Is it okay to take this supplement?
    (Bring any workout supplements you are taking to your doctor visits. Many pre-workout drinks can raise blood pressure, and many post-workout drinks have ingredients that can affect blood sugar.)
4. What can I take for this injury? (If you do have musculoskeletal pain, ask your doctor before taking over-the-counter medications like Motrin (ibuprofen) or Aleve (naproxen) for any extended period of time. These nonsteroidal anti-inflammatory drugs (NSAIDs) can cause irritation to the stomach and damage to the kidneys, and over time can increase the risk for heart problems.)

Notes

1. L. Byberg et al., "Total Mortality After Changes in Leisure Time Physical Activity in 50 Year Old Men: 35 Year Follow-up of Population Based Cohort," *BMJ* 338 (2009): b688, doi: 10.1136/bmj.b688.
2. S. La Vignera et al., "Statins and Erectile Dysfunction: A Critical Summary of Current Evidence," *Journal of Andrology* 33, no. 4 (2012): 552–558, doi: 10.2164/jandrol.111.015230.
3. J. B. Gillen et al., "Twelve Weeks of Sprint Interval Training Improves Indices of Cardiometabolic Health Similar to Traditional Endurance Training Despite a Five-Fold Lower Exercise Volume and Time Commitment," *PLoS One* 11, no. 4 (2016): e0154075, doi: 10.1371/journal.pone.0154075.

4. G. E. Orer and N. A. Guzel, "The Effects of Acute L-Carnitine Supplementation on Endurance Performance of Athletes," *Journal of Strength and Conditioning Research* 28, no. 2 (2014): 514–519, doi: 10.1519/JSC.0b013e3182a76790.

5. D. K. Eaton et al., "Youth Risk Behavior Surveillance—United States, 2009," *Morbidity and Mortality Weekly Report: Surveillance Summaries* 59 (2010): 16.

6. M. A. Tahririan et al., "Ultrasound Guided Platelet-Rich Plasma Injection for the Treatment of Rotator Cuff Tendinopathy," *Advanced Biomedical Research* 5 (2016): 200, doi: 10.4103/2277-9175.190939.

7. M. T. Jensen et al., "Elevated Resting Heart Rate, Physical Fitness and All-Cause Mortality: A 16-Year Follow-up in the Copenhagen Male Study," *Heart* 99 (2013): 882–887, doi: 10.1136/heartjnl-2012-303375.

8. R. Ross et al., "Importance of Assessing Cardiorespiratory Fitness in Clinical Practice: A Case for Fitness as a Clinical Vital Sign: A Scientific Statement from the American Heart Association," *Circulation* 134, no. 24 (2016): e653–e699, doi: 10.1161/CIR.0000000000000461.

Resources

HeartMath is a nonprofit that leads the way in measuring heart rate variability, one of the best measures of stress and strain from your sympathetic nervous system: www.heartmath.com/innerbalance.
At-home workouts:

- NerdFitness (www.nerdfitness.com) is a great online community for regular guys looking to get more fit. It has an active online community, good tips, and an online coaching program that can work with anyone at any level for home-based or gym-based workouts.
- *Men's Journal* magazine has a great website, including tips for in-home workouts: https://www.mensjournal.com/health-fitness/10-home-workouts-build-muscle-under-20-minutes.
- Beachbody (www.beachbody.com) is one of the leaders in at-home workout programs, famous for its P90X program. The company is constantly updating its programs, but get a clearance from your doctor before starting any—they can be intense.
- The Men's Fitness channel on YouTube has a "Today's Workout" series that is great for beginners, as it shows proper form for various exercises.

https://www.youtube.com/watch?v=WWJww0G6Aq4

14

Optimal Aging

The first thing you'll notice about this chapter is that its title is "Optimal Aging" and not "Antiaging." There are a lot of services and products, from hormones to supplements to plastic surgery, that promise to stop or reverse the aging process. This chapter will attempt to separate the hype from the reality when it comes to what you can do not just to potentially add years to your life but also, and just as important, to minimize age-related physical decline and the associated health risks. I'll cover the lifestyle habits that potentially can add years to your life and the top supplements that help attenuate the effects of aging on the body, and I'll offer a few words about the use of hormones.

Lifestyle Habits

The five habits that are most strongly associated with a longer life span may not be surprising, but the impact of these five is likely greater than you realize. A recent study using data on over 100,000 people from the Nurses' Health Study and the Health Professionals' Follow-up Study showed that maintaining these habits can add twelve years to a fifty-year old's life span, compared to a similar individual who has none of these habits. What are they?

1. Not smoking cigarettes
2. Maintaining a healthy weight
3. Regular physical activity
4. Moderate alcohol intake
5. Eating a healthy diet

See? If you've read this far in the book, you won't be surprised that these habits are good for you. But adding an average of twelve years is more than anyone would have thought! Without any of these habits, a fifty-year-old American man has a life expectancy of 25.5 more years—that is, on average he'll live until he's over 75. With all five, that same man can be expected to live 37.6 more years, until he's over 87.[1]

I mentioned the Blue Zones in Chapter 6—those regions of the world where people live longer and healthier than anywhere else on earth, as discovered and written about by *National Geographic* journalist Dan Buettner. In his book *The Blue Zones*, he describes how he set out to find the lifestyle habits prevalent in those societies with the highest proportions of centenarians (people who live to be over a hundred years old).[2] The habits they share fall largely into these same categories as the five I've just mentioned (see also Box 6.1 in Chapter 6).[3]

Let's take a closer look at these categories of behaviors. Not smoking is clear-cut, but what specifically does it mean to have regular physical activity, maintain a healthy weight, drink moderate amounts of alcohol, and eat a healthy diet? By drilling down a little deeper, we can know how best to claim those twelve extra years for ourselves.

Physical Activity

Regular physical activity is generally defined as more than thirty minutes a day of moderate or vigorous activity (including brisk walking). But older people in these Blue Zones don't necessarily engage in defined periods of exercise. It seems that being physically active in general is what's important—taking the stairs instead of the elevator, walking a few blocks extra, and riding a bicycle for transportation all count as the type of regular physical activity needed to add healthy years to your life.

Healthy Weight

A healthy weight was defined in the study about life span as a body mass index (BMI) above 18.5 and under 25. Obesity is associated with so many of the diseases of aging (especially diabetes, heart disease, and hypertension) that maintaining a healthy weight contributes to longevity by decreasing risk for these diseases. However, waist circumference predicts heart attack risk better than BMI. Men with a waist size larger than 40 inches have significantly increased risk for heart disease and diabetes.

Moderate Alcohol Consumption

Moderate alcohol consumption is defined as up to two drinks per day, with a drink being 1½ ounces of hard liquor, 6 ounces of wine, or 12 ounces of beer. In fact, studies show that not drinking alcohol at all is not as good for longevity as drinking a moderate amount, most likely because of the beneficial effect on heart disease and stroke risk from one to two drinks per day for men. But having more than two drinks per day on a regular basis contributes to health problems such as liver disease, auto accidents, and increased risk of certain cancers.

Eating a Healthy Diet

In the studies on life expectancy, what counts as a healthy diet lines up fairly well with what the Blue Zones regions have in common in terms of diet—basically, what we've calling an anti-inflammatory or Mediterranean-style diet. Chapter 2 goes into detail on this type of diet, but broadly speaking, it consists of:

- Emphasis on plants: fruits, vegetables, legumes, seeds, nuts
- Lean animal protein with some but not all meals
- Whole, unrefined grains
- Reasonable portion size: an average plate might have 6 ounces of animal protein (about the size of your fist), 1 cup of whole grains, and the rest loaded with vegetables
- Minimal refined sugar

Optimal Aging

- Minimal processed foods (foods that need to be manufactured rather than raised or grown)
- No trans fats (such as hydrogenated oils)
- Healthier monounsaturated or polyunsaturated fats from olives, nuts, avocados, fish, seeds, and legumes

There's a lot of evidence showing that eating fewer calories leads to a longer life. Approaches such as intermittent fasting (when you restrict all eating to a narrow window, such as eight or nine hours, during any twenty-four-hour period) and complete fasting one day a week are still being investigated. Other studies show the antiaging effects of intermittent fasting. For example, a study from the Harvard School of Public Health showed how periodic fasting can help our energy-producing mitochondria to function better as we age.[4]

One interesting approach has been developed by Valter Longo, an expert in biology and aging at the University of Southern California's Davis School of Gerontology. The diet described in his book *The Longevity Diet* mimics the effect of fasting on the body with a fasting-mimicking diet periodically done for five days on top of a general eating regimen that is largely vegan, with some fish, and lower amounts of protein than many people feel they need. I am intrigued by the research he describes showing the diet's positive effect on the body in terms of decreased inflammation and improvement in autoimmune diseases.[5]

Purpose

The other aspect of living that Dan Buettner pointed out from his research on the Blue Zones is that most members of these communities are clear about their purpose—the reason they get up in the morning. He was able to calculate that the simple act of clearly identifying a sense of purpose was associated with an additional seven years of life expectancy.

This sense of purpose can be a specific goal, such as getting a promotion at work, or it can be a general sense of what you want to accomplish over the next few years. It can also be about connecting deeply with others or with a higher power. In Japan the concept of *ikigai* is defined as a reason for getting up in the morning. Figure 14.1 shows especially well what is meant by *ikigai*. Your purpose can change over time, but having some sort of overarching goal seems to activate internal mechanisms that help you to be more resilient and active.

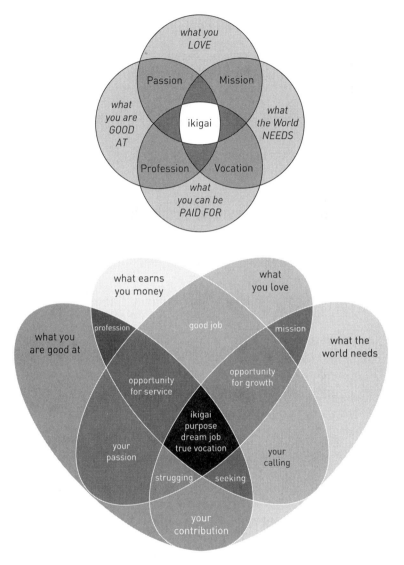

Figure 14.1 Ikigai

Source: Alex Myles, "Discover Your Ikigai—Your Reason for Living," *Elephant Journal*, March 29, 2016, https://www.elephantjournal.com/2016/03/discover-your-ikigai-your-reason-for-living.

Supplements

There are supplements that can be helpful in slowing down the impact of aging on the body. Some of them have been discussed in Chapter 4, but it's worth mentioning here my top recommendations for managing the aging process.

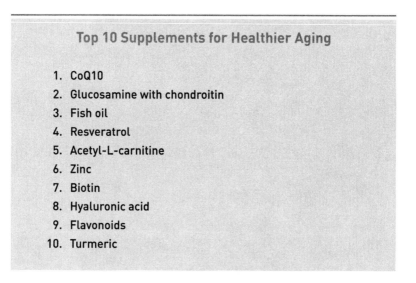

Top 10 Supplements for Healthier Aging

1. CoQ10
2. Glucosamine with chondroitin
3. Fish oil
4. Resveratrol
5. Acetyl-L-carnitine
6. Zinc
7. Biotin
8. Hyaluronic acid
9. Flavonoids
10. Turmeric

1. CoQ10 (Coenzyme Q10)

This antioxidant has proven to be particularly beneficial for boosting energy production on a cellular level as well as improving the appearance of aging skin. A 2016 study found an association between taking 150 mg of CoQ10 daily for twelve weeks and reduced wrinkles around the eyes and mouth, compared to the use of a placebo.[6] CoQ10 is found naturally in organ meats, beef, and mackerel, and to a lesser extent in spinach, broccoli, and cauliflower. But for the most noticeable effects on energy and skin, you'll have to take a supplement.

2. Glucosamine and Chondroitin

Glucosamine, extracted from shellfish like crab and lobster, can minimize the achiness that comes from age-related arthritis, especially when combined with chondroitin, which is a natural component of cartilage. If your joints are getting achy, I recommend trying these supplements at doses of 1,000 mg glucosamine with 400–500 mg chondroitin. Give these a couple of months to have an effect, but if you don't notice any improvement in pain by then, I'd recommend stopping them.

3. Fish Oil

The omega-3-fatty acids EPA and DHA are possibly the most important weapon we have to ward off the effects of aging. These substances are potent anti-inflammatory compounds, act as mild blood thinners to help prevent clots, improve mood, and lower LDL ("bad" cholesterol). People with the highest levels of omega-3 fatty acids showed the least shortening of telomeres, one measure of biological aging (discussed later in this chapter).[7] Those with the lowest levels of omega-3s had the fastest rate of telomere shortening. The recommended dose is generally 2,000 mg per day of EPA and DHA combined. You can also get omega-3s in supplements made from algae. Food sources of omega-3 fatty acids are flaxseed, walnuts, dark green leafy vegetables, and even eggs, but the ability to convert the omega-3s in these sources to EPA and DHA varies from person to person.

4. Resveratrol

This compound, found in red wine, is sometimes called the "longevity molecule" because it has been shown to lengthen the life span of many different animal species. Research also suggests resveratrol can help prevent several diseases related to aging, including diabetes, Alzheimer's, and heart disease.[8] Resveratrol can be taken as a supplement, but there is a similar supplement, pterostilbene, that seems to be more bioavailable (easily absorbed and utilized in the body). I recommend 50 mg a day of pterostilbene to help unlock longevity molecules called sirtuins, as discussed in Chapter 12.

5. Acetyl-L-Carnitine

A dose of 1,000 mg of acetyl-L-carnitine every day can improve your cells' ability to make energy, translating to more overall energy for living your life. In addition, it can help keep you sharp as you get older. Make sure to get the acetyl form, and not just plain L-carnitine, in order to get beneficial neurological effects. Food sources are mostly animal-based foods such as poultry, milk, and meat.

6. Zinc

This essential trace mineral plays a role in maintaining normal testosterone levels, prostate health, immune function, cell division, and wound healing. I recommend supplementing with 20 mg, along with 2 mg of copper to keep the body's natural ratio of the two minerals at 10:1. Meat, nuts, and legumes (especially hemp seeds) are good food sources of zinc. Most men's multivitamins will have zinc because of its crucial role in men's health.

7. Biotin

Supplementing with this B vitamin is recommended for healthy skin and hair, both of which tend to lose their luster as we age. Supplementing with biotin also may help regulate blood sugar levels in people with type 2 diabetes. Good food sources of biotin include eggs, mushrooms, cauliflower, and almonds. I recommend supplementing with 50 mcg a day.

8. Hyaluronic Acid

This clear fluid, found in your skin, joints, and other body tissues, helps retain moisture and keeps things flexible. Since a lack of synovial fluid—of which hyaluronic acid is a component—in the joints can lead to painful stiffening, supplementing with hyaluronic acid may help relieve these symptoms. A 2016 data review examining the effects of hyaluronic acid on knee pain found that hyaluronic acid supplements "provide at least some possibility for the treatment and prevention of serious conditions in patients with osteoarthritis exhibiting mild knee pain."[9] Hyaluronic acid's strong moisture-retaining properties also make it a popular skin care ingredient in moisturizers. Topical use with a product containing at least

0.1 percent hyaluronic acid may help skin elasticity and reduce the appearance of wrinkles.

9. Flavonoids

These phytonutrients, found in fruits, vegetables, and tea, have powerful antioxidant and anti-inflammatory powers. In addition to reducing your risk of heart disease and other chronic health concerns, flavonoids may help prevent the weight gain that often comes with aging. One study of 124,000 people showed that those with the highest flavonoid intake gained the least amount of weight as they aged.[10] And a twenty-year Harvard University study showed that men who ate flavonoid-rich foods three times a week experienced less erectile dysfunction as they aged.[11] Foods high in flavonoids include black tea, citrus fruits, berries, and most green and red vegetables. You can take a supplement with a complex of flavonoids to augment your intake.

10. Turmeric

Turmeric is a popular supplement because it contains a powerfully anti-inflammatory and antioxidant active constituent called curcumin. Among many other applications, turmeric has been shown to help reduce symptoms of arthritis. In an Italian study of patients with osteoarthritis in one or both knees, those who took a turmeric formulation for ninety days showed a 58 percent reduction in overall pain and stiffness compared to controls. They were also able to reduce their need for painkillers such as aspirin and ibuprofen by 63 percent compared to patients on conventional medical therapy alone.[12] I generally recommend a dose of 1,000 mg turmeric that includes black pepper to help with absorption. Turmeric is gaining popularity as a topical antiaging ingredient as well; moisturizers containing turmeric extract have been shown to improve the appearance of fine lines, wrinkles, and age spots.

Hormones

Maintaining healthy hormone levels is crucial to minimize age-related cellular and tissue damage. This includes thyroid hormones, cortisol (our main stress hormone), insulin and leptin (hormones that affect blood sugar and hunger), and the sex hormones, testosterone and estrogen. Low testosterone is associated with accelerated loss of muscle mass, which can accelerate physical aging. Testosterone supplementation may combat immunosenescence, age-related changes in immune cells that can lead to inflammation and increased infection risk. It's important to have your free testosterone checked, as the protein that binds testosterone (sex hormone binding globulin, SHBG) can increase with age, making the total testosterone level normal while most is bound up with SHBG and unavailable to do its work. Measuring free hormone levels gives a more accurate picture of true bioavailable testosterone. I recommend having the following hormones tested at least yearly in order to make sure they are all optimized, as both low and high levels can be stressful on the body as it ages.

- Testosterone, total and free
- Estrogen (yes, even in men)
- TSH, free T3, and free T4 (thyroid hormones)
- Morning cortisol, or salivary cortisol measured four times over the course of one day
- Fasting insulin
- Leptin

If any of these hormones are off, you need to get them back into balance. Hormones by definition have effects all over the body, so abnormal levels of any of them will affect overall metabolism and inflammation, key processes in aging. For example, thyroid hormones are master hormones for hair growth, metabolism and calorie-burning, sleep, and temperature regulation. The incidence of hypothyroidism (low thyroid hormone activity) increases with age, and the symptoms of low thyroid mimic many symptoms of aging: mental slowness, constipation, weight gain, and fatigue. Cortisol can be reduced to abnormally low levels by chronic stress or chronic illness, and too-low cortisol also causes low energy and depression. The most important thing to keep in mind about hormones is that they all work together—finely tuned in health, but causing a cascade of problems when not optimized. Their interactions necessitate looking at all of them because, like an orchestra, if one is off, the whole performance is affected.

A Word on Human Growth Hormone (HGH)

Produced by your pituitary gland, natural growth hormone propels our childhood development and helps with cell growth as well as organ and tissue function throughout our entire lives. Because our bodies make less growth hormone as we age, some people turn to synthetic human growth hormone (HGH) in an attempt to slow the aging process. The makers of HGH claim it can increase muscle mass, boost libido, and improve energy levels—essentially turn back the clock. But human growth hormone comes with high costs, both physiological and financial.

HGH is only FDA-approved to be used by adults for a handful of reasons, including pituitary deficiencies caused by tumors and muscle-wasting disease associated with HIV/AIDS. This means the vast majority of people using human growth hormone are using it for other, unsanctioned reasons. Athletes and bodybuilders hoping to enhance performance may turn to doctors who are willing to prescribe human growth hormone off-label for unapproved purposes. Others hoping to reverse the aging process may obtain HGH from online pharmacies, websites, or antiaging "clinics" claiming their product does everything from regrow hair to enhance memory, but many of these promises are unfounded. Research shows that HGH does increase lean muscle mass and energy levels while reducing body fat. However, it also causes a range of side effects such as joint pain, carpal tunnel syndrome, edema, and potential for an increase in both blood sugar and cancer risk.

In a review of forty-four studies looking at the effects of human growth hormone on athletes, 303 volunteers were given daily HGH injections, while 137 others received placebo shots. After around twenty days, the HGH group saw significant gains in lean body mass—an average of 4.6 pounds. But the additional mass didn't lead to improved performance, with the HGH group showing no increase in strength or exercise capacity. And those who received HGH were more likely than the placebo group to retain fluid and experience fatigue.[13]

Most users of HGH report a high rate of side effects, including fluid retention, breast enlargement, and joint pain. Furthermore, there is research suggesting HGH may increase the risk of cancer in general and prostate cancer in particular. The concern is that cancer cells are, by definition, growing rapidly. We all have cancer cells that pop up now and then, but our immune system generally takes care of them. If we artificially raise the level of growth hormone in our bodies, this could stimulate the growth of such cancer cells over and above what the immune system can handle. This risk has not yet been confirmed in studies, but the possibility should serve as a caution about the potential long-term risks of off-label use.

Pharmaceutical HGH itself is a subcutaneous injection that costs well over $1,000 a week. There are a lot of fake HGH products out there— sublingual and oral formulations—that have not been shown to be effective and may contain dangerous ingredients, some of which aren't even disclosed on the packaging. There are many companies and websites that have been called out by the FDA for making unsubstantiated claims.

So while HGH is effective in specific areas, including increasing lean muscle mass, it comes with serious risk. Is it really worth the financial cost and the side effects, not to mention the potential risk of cancer? One way to boost your own natural production of HGH is to work on your sleep. We make most of our HGH when we sleep, so increasing the hours and quality of your sleep can augment your levels naturally.

STAN WANTS TO STAY FEELING YOUNG

Most of my patients who come to me for an optimal health program are between forty and sixty-five, anxious to make sure they are doing all they can to stay healthy and prevent diseases from interfering with their busy lives. But Stan was different. He was a retired seventy-two-year-old who had recently started a relationship with a fifty-three-year-old. It was getting serious, and Stan wanted to make sure their time together was full of adventure and fun, not caretaking and doctor visits. He wanted to know what he could do to stay as healthy and vibrant as possible for as long as possible. Testing and his personal medical history didn't reveal any potential roadblocks to this, so we set about to make an overall blueprint for Stan to stay vital.

I recommended he eat a pescatarian diet (a vegetarian diet that also includes fish) and restricting his eating to eight hours out of each day. He chose to eat his first meal around noon, allowing him to have dinner at seven o'clock and finish by eight. We started him on an exercise program that included yoga (for balance, fall prevention, flexibility, strength, and nervous system relaxation), weight training once a week, and cardio on a treadmill twice a week.

We added some of the supplements mentioned in this chapter and Chapter 12, including NAD with pterostilbene, a joint support formula, and acetyl-L-carnitine. Lastly, we made sure his sleep was restful and of adequate duration by using some meditation practices before bed along with melatonin.

Stan followed the whole program religiously, felt great, and was happy to be so proactive. The funny thing is that he felt better than his younger partner, who was a little overweight and was starting to have some joint pain and blood sugar issues. Stan brought his partner in to see me, insisting they do the whole plan together.

Measuring Physical Aging

So how can we measure aging—specifically, how much impact the passage of time is having on our physical bodies? One way is through looking at how our cells are aging. We can do this by looking at telomeres. Telomeres are the ends of the DNA strands in our cells. In order to make new cells, DNA needs to make a copy of itself, and every time it does that, the ends need to be kept from fraying. Telomeres protect those ends but get shorter over time. When they get sufficiently short, the cell stops dividing efficiently and is more prone to dying. The longer our telomeres, the more times our cells can multiply in healthy ways, and the lower our risk of getting age-related illness. Geneticists have found that people with short telomeres die sooner. Now telomere length can be measured with a simple blood test, as a sort of measure of biological (as opposed to chronological) age.

Telomere shortening can be the result of the same processes that make us age more rapidly—basically anything that causes acute or chronic in-flammation. One study looked at telomere length in white blood cells on two occasions five years apart. Those with the lowest levels of the anti-inflammatory fats EPA and DHA had more than two and a half times the rate of telomere shortening as those with the highest amounts.[14] In another study, telomeres were longer in those who were active as opposed to those who were sedentary. Genetic factors and environmental factors can also affect the length of the telomere. It has even been shown that overall fitness is correlated with telomere length.

The Bottom Line

The strategies mentioned in this chapter provide a powerful blueprint for minimizing the effect of aging. In Table 14.1 I offer a sample "antiaging" week that incorporates many of the proven tools mentioned here. Take a look and modify it to fit your own schedule, interests, and goals. Most of all, realize that through lifestyle, hormone optimization, and supplements, you have more control over the effects of aging than you might have realized.

Sunday: Think about your purpose. Studies show that people who have a clearly identified sense of purpose have a life expectancy up to seven years longer.

Monday: How was your sleep last night? Inadequate sleep accelerates oxidative stress and speeds up aging. Tonight, try getting at least seven hours of sleep. Keep your cellphone or iPad out of your bedroom tonight. Cover any electronics that have blue LED lights. Before bed, have some chamomile tea.

Tuesday: Stress is toxic to the brain. High cortisol levels damage neurons and accelerate brain aging. Evoking the relaxation response protects the brain from these toxic effects of stress, and the most powerful way to evoke that response is with meditation. Download the 10%

Table 14.1 Antiaging Week

Sunday	Monday	Tuesday	Wednesday	Thursday	Friday	Saturday
Write down your thoughts about your purpose.	Sleep at least 7 hours.	Meditate for 20 minutes.	Sugar-free day.	Physical activity: hike, bike, swim, walk, or run.	Have a glass of wine.	Spend time with friends.

Happier app or something similar (see Chapter 6) and try a twenty-minute meditation.

Wednesday: Today is a sugar-free day. Besides being a factor in weight gain, sugar causes inflammation, a process that is the common denominator behind many diseases of aging. Skip the sweetener in your coffee and grab fruit instead of a muffin for breakfast. Avoid white bread, white potatoes, and white pasta, as these foods are rich in simple carbohydrates, which act a lot like plain sugar in the body. Instead, have salads with a protein or a quinoa bowl.

Thursday: Start moving. Once a week is not enough, but it's a start. Engage in at least one hour of physical activity today. You can hike, walk, run, swim, or go for a bike ride. Don't forget to warm up with a gradual increase in intensity for the first ten minutes, and save the last ten minutes for a cool-down. Stretch afterward.

Friday: It's time to have a glass of wine. Yes, unless you have issues with alcohol, a glass of wine in the evening is a habit enjoyed by many residents of the Blue Zones.

Saturday: Spend time with friends. Social interaction is key to a long life, and social isolation is as a strong a risk factor for early death as smoking.

Questions to Ask Your Doctor

1. Are these symptoms normal? (Don't simply chalk up any physical symptoms to "old age." You can reverse many aches and pains, weight gain, and fatigue with proper treatment of medical conditions and changes in diet or lifestyle as described in this chapter. Ask your doctor about any symptoms that are interfering with your quality of life.)

2. Is there anything I need to be cautious about regarding exercise? (Ask if you have any limitations to exercise, and then get started on a program that keeps you active.)

Notes

1. Y. Li et al., "Impact of Healthy Lifestyle Factors on Life Expectancies in the US Population," *Circulation* 138 (2018): 345–355, doi: 10.1161/CIRCULATIONAHA.117.032047.

2. The five Blue Zones regions are Sardinia, Italy; Ikaria, Greece; Okinawa, Japan; Loma Linda, California; and Nicoya Peninsula, Costa Rica.
3. To sum up the information in Box 6.1, this is what people in the Blue Zones have in common:

    1. Clear identification of a sense of overall purpose
    2. Regular physical activity
    3. Active management and reduction of stress
    4. 80% rule: stop eating when you're 80% full
    5. Eating more plants and less meat
    6. Having some sort of spiritual practice
    7. Caring for and feeling cared for by loved ones

4. Karen Feldscher, "In Pursuit of Healthy Aging: Harvard Study Shows How Intermittent Fasting and Manipulating Mitochondrial Networks May Increase Lifespan," *Harvard Gazette*, November 3, 2017, https://news.harvard.edu/gazette/story/2017/11/intermittent-fasting-may-be-center-of-increasing-lifespan.
5. I. Y. Choi et al., "Diet Mimicking Fasting Promotes Regeneration and Reduces Autoimmunity and Multiple Sclerosis Symptoms," *Cell Reports* 15, no. 10 (2016): 2136–2146, doi:10.1016/j.celrep.2016.05.009.
6. K. Žmitek et al., "The Effect of Dietary Intake of Coenzyme Q10 on Skin Parameters and Condition: Results of a Randomized, Placebo-Controlled, Double-Blind Study," *BioFactors* 43 (2017): 132–140, doi:10.1002/biof.1316.
7. R. Farzaneh-Far et al., "Association of Marine Omega-3 Fatty Acid Levels with Telomeric Aging in Patients with Coronary Heart Disease," *Journal of the American Medical Association* 303, no. 3 (2010): 250–257, doi: 10.1001/jama.2009.2008.
8. B. P. Hubbard et al., "Evidence for a Common Mechanism of SIRT1 Regulation by Allosteric Activators," *Science* 339, no. 6124 (2013): 1216–1219, doi: 10.1126/science.1231097.
9. M. Oe et al., "Oral Hyaluronan Relieves Knee Pain: A Review," *Nutrition Journal* 15, no. 11 (2016), doi:10.1186/s12937-016-0128-2.
10. M. L. Bertoia et al., "Dietary Flavonoid Intake and Weight Maintenance: Three Prospective Cohorts of 124,086 US Men and Women Followed for Up to 24 Years," *BMJ* 28, no. 352 (2016): i17, doi: 10.1136/bmj.i17.
11. A. Cassidy et al., "Dietary Flavonoid Intake and Incidence of Erectile Dysfunction," *American Journal of Clinical Nutrition* 103, no. 2 (2016): 534–541, doi: 10.3945/ajcn.115.122010.

12. G. Belcaro et al., "Product-Evaluation Registry of Meriva®, Curcumin-Phosphatidylcholine Complex, for the Complementary Management of Osteoarthritis," *Panminerva Medica* 52, no. 2 supp. 1 (2010): 55–62.

13. H. Liu et al., "Systematic Review: The Effects of Growth Hormone on Athletic Performance," *Annals of Internal Medicine* 148, no. 10 (2008): 747–758.

14. R. Farzaneh-Far et al., "Association of Marine Omega-3 Fatty Acid Levels with Telomeric Aging in Patients with Coronary Heart Disease," *Journal of the American Medical Association* 303, no. 3 (2010): 250–257, doi: 10.1001/jama.2009.2008.

Resources

The nine commonalities of populations in the Blue Zones: https://www.bluezones.com/2016/11/power-9.

On intermittent fasting: One of the articles that got the intermittent fasting craze started is from *Scientific American*, https://www.scientificamerican.com/article/how-intermittent-fasting-might-help-you-live-longer-healthier-life. Also see *The Scientific Approach to Intermittent Fasting* by Michael VanDerschelden (2016).

SECTION 3

Complementary Medicine and Men's Health

15

Traditional Chinese Medicine for Men

When you hear about traditional Chinese medicine (TCM), you may think of acupuncture. But TCM involves much more than acupuncture; it is a complete system of medicine that dates back at least 2,500 years, with some experts estimating it was practiced as long as 5,000 years ago. While there are many aspects to it, in general it is based on the following ideas:

- Each person possesses a vital energy, known as qi, that supports health and performs critical functions as it flows through the body. Your qi is believed to wane as you age.
- Health is a state that occurs when two opposing yet complementary forces, yin and yang, are in harmony. When the balance between these two forces is thrown off, illness results.
- Everything that happens, in the body as well as in the larger world, can be symbolized and/or explained by the five elements: fire, earth, wood, metal, and water. Different organs of the body are associated with different elements. The heart and small intestine are under the fire element; earth includes the stomach and spleen; the liver and gallbladder

are associated with wood; the lungs and large intestine belong with metal; and the water element includes the bladder and kidneys.

- Illness is caused by blockages in flow of energy. Channels (called "meridians" in TCM) are pathways of qi flow that can be blocked, causing "stagnation" in organs or in the meridians that can cause symptoms or disease. Such blockages can be treated with needles (acupuncture), movement (qi gong, tai chi), herbs, suction (cupping), burning of mugwort near the channels (moxibustion), and manual therapies such as massage (twina) or vigorous rubbing (gwasha).

TCM is a broad modality with its own system of medical diagnosis and many different types of interventions. Practitioners attend at least four years of rigorous graduate-level training to become doctors of Chinese medicine, then take additional exams in order to be licensed or certified. Only three states in the United States have no provision for licensure in TCM.

Chinese medical diagnosis usually involves the practitioner checking the pulse or examining the tongue to infer where there is disturbance in the qi or imbalance among the five elements. This system of diagnosis and treatment is very different from what we are used to in Western medicine, but it been around for millennia and is backed up not just by experience but also by high-quality research, even if we Westerners can't fully understand how it works. In this chapter, I will review some specific TCM approaches to conditions of interest to men.

Mitch: TCM for a Triathlete

Mitch was training for a triathlon. He'd been feeling great, but overdid it when he did a trial swim-bike-run one weekend, and he came in complaining of some ankle pain. He didn't break or seriously tear anything, but the mild sprain was limiting his training and threatening his ability to be ready for the big race. In addition to taking anti-inflammatories, he wanted to know what else he could do to recover and minimize his pain.

I recommended Mitch see a TCM practitioner. When he was examined, the practitioner looked at his tongue to see if it was swollen, had a coating, or had cracks in it. All of these features give clues about blocked channels or imbalances between yin and yang. The practitioner also checked his pulses—but very differently than I would do, by checking pulses on both wrists in three different locations and at various depths. This helped to determine if Mitch was depleted or suffering from other imbalances—between hot and cold or dampness and dryness, for example. This tongue and pulse examination, along with his symptoms, helped the TCM expert understand what organs were out of balance and what channels were blocked, leading to his pain. The practitioner treated the imbalance and blockage with a dozen tiny needles, so small that Mitch could barely feel them go in. The needles stayed in for about twenty minutes each session, and Mitch found this time extremely relaxing—he even drifted off to sleep during a couple of the sessions. After each treatment, his pain got better, until it was completely relieved after six treatments.

Acupuncture

Acupuncture uses extremely fine needles placed in specific positions along meridians. The exact placement depends on the imbalance or condition being treated. Like other pillars of TCM, acupuncture has been practiced for thousands of years. It started to gain momentum in the United States in the early 1970s, when President Nixon began opening up relations with China. In 1971, just a day after Secretary of State Henry Kissinger made a secret visit to China, a New York Times journalist in China, James Reston, required emergency surgery for appendicitis. Acupuncture was used to relieve his pain after the surgery. Reston wrote about his experience for the newspaper, just as America was becoming more interested in Chinese culture as a whole.

Because there is such strong evidence of the value of acupuncture to treat conditions ranging from autoimmune disease to pain, it is now used at academic medical centers like Harvard, UCLA, and Johns Hopkins. It's also very popular in Europe and elsewhere around the world. Acupuncture has become one of the most extensively researched alternative healing practices—a simple search in a research database yields thousands of studies involving acupuncture.

Acupuncture is exceptionally helpful as a complementary therapy, meaning it can be used alongside other, more conventional forms of treatment. It's most commonly used for pain (back pain, arthritis, and other musculoskeletal pain especially), but it has several other applications.

What exactly happens during an acupuncture treatment may vary depending on the practitioner. Typically, the initial evaluation will involve an examination of your pulse in multiple places along both wrists and an assessment of your tongue. Based on these findings, the practitioner will determine which acupuncture points along which meridians should be treated. Generally, there may be insertion of between five and twenty needles, which are so thin they usually don't cause discomfort going in. Gentle manipulation of the needles may include twirling, application of heat, or mild electrical pulses while you lie still and relax with the needles in place for ten to twenty minutes. Many people find the whole experience extremely relaxing.

Because it can be a powerful therapy, acupuncture has gained much respect in the mainstream medical community. The United States military has even started using acupuncture to treat pain both in the field (using a special technique of acupuncture on various points on the ear, called battlefield acupuncture) and at military medical centers, and studies show it may also be useful for easing the symptoms of post-traumatic stress disorder (PTSD).[1],[2]

How could this possibly work? Currently the most accepted theory of the mechanism of acupuncture is that the stimulation activates the fascia network, an idea similar to the meridian theory of TCM. Research has shown that sticking a needle into a point along a meridian does cause changes in activity in the part of the brain TCM considers connected to that meridian, whereas inserting a needle away from that meridian doesn't have the same impact.[3] Acupuncture is very safe. The most common side effects include local pain from needling and slight bleeding, but that is rare. The World Health Organization reports that the incidence of serious adverse events from acupuncture is 0.024 percent.

Who Can Benefit from Acupuncture?

Acupuncture is a therapy that involves the insertion of hair-thin needles at specific points on the body. Men experiencing the following conditions may find acupuncture helpful when used as a complement to conventional treatment:

- High blood pressure
- Prostatitis
- Prostate cancer
- Addiction
- Erectile dysfunction
- Premature ejaculation
- Infertility
- Back pain
- Insomnia
- Sports injuries and muscle soreness

Chinese Herbal Medicine

As with other systems of healing used around the globe, herbs are an important part of TCM. Unfortunately, many herbs imported from China are contaminated with toxins, heavy metals, or pharmaceuticals, or are mislabeled. So it is important to seek guidance from a professional before taking Chinese herbs. Some of the better-quality brands are sourced from Taiwan or the United States. Here are some of the more widely used Chinese herbs.

Astragalus

This root is prized for its tonifying ability, particularly when it comes to strengthening the immune system. You can usually find sliced astragalus root at health food stores, and it can also be taken in capsule form.

It is often used in formulas that are helpful in preventing or treating viral infections.

Ginseng

There are actually several species called ginseng, but Asian (or Korean) ginseng (*Panax ginseng*) is especially good for brain function (memory, concentration) and general physical endurance. Ginseng is probably the most well-known Chinese herb, and it's used by herbalists and other practitioners the world over. Revered in TCM for its ability to boost one's qi, this fortifying, tonic herb is helpful for a huge array of conditions. (I'll get to ginseng's use for sexual dysfunction soon.)

In Chinese medicine, American ginseng (*Panax quinquefolius*) is considered cooling and calming, whereas Asian ginseng is more stimulating. Siberian ginseng (*Eleutherococcus senticosus*) is actually a different species of plant entirely and is useful in boosting the immune system.

Licorice

This root is a popular ingredient in many herbal formulas due to its relatively sweet taste. It's often used in the West to soothe sore throats, and some people even chew on pieces of licorice root to help them quit smoking. Licorice can help with gastrointestinal reflux, but it can raise blood pressure because it contains a substance called glycyrrhizin. So I often recommend deglycyrrhizinated licorice, or DGL, for this condition.

Combination Herbal Formulas

In addition to single Chinese herbs, many TCM practitioners will recommend combination formulas sold as pills, syrups, creams, and other easy-to-use preparations. Commonly referred to as Chinese patent remedies, these formulas can be purchased at some health food stores and, of course, online.

Bi Yan Pian

This combination is frequently recommended for sinus congestion, pressure, and pain. It can be especially helpful for those struggling with seasonal allergies.

Yin Chiao

One of the most popular patent formulas, this one is good for relieving cold and flu symptoms, especially when it's taken during the first day or two of illness.

Bai Hua Yu

Also known as white flower oil, this topical analgesic can help relieve muscle pain caused by overexertion. Some people even call this one the "Chinese Bengay."

Tai Chi and Qi Gong

You may have seen images of groups of people moving in synchronized choreographed ways in parks in China or Chinatowns across North America. Sometimes referred to as "meditation in motion" because of its graceful movements and emphasis on deep breathing, tai chi was originally developed as a form of self-defense but has become instead an extremely gentle means of mindful exercise. This low-impact practice is considered safe enough for people of all ages and abilities, and it may be particularly beneficial for older adults because it can improve balance. It is a little like self-acupuncture, because the movements in tai chi help to improve the flow of qi throughout the system. Tai chi has even been shown to help manage the symptoms of congestive heart failure.

Qi gong is very similar to tai chi in that it emphasizes slow, deliberate movements and breathing techniques. Individual movements and accompanying breath work or meditations may be practiced to manage specific symptoms or conditions independently or in a group, or as prescribed by a TCM practitioner.

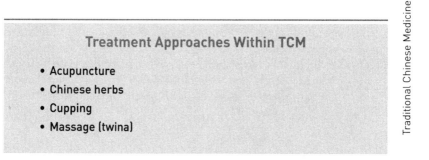

Treatment Approaches Within TCM

- Acupuncture
- Chinese herbs
- Cupping
- Massage (twina)

- Nutrition based on Chinese medicine diagnosis
- Tai chi and qi gong
- Vigorous rubbing by the practitioner (gwasha)

The Benefits of TCM Specifically in Men's Health

You may be thinking that TCM is only for pain or for those wanting to avoid Western medications. Actually, there are many health issues relevant to men that TCM can help with, either as an adjunct to Western medicine or in place of it. Because it is such an entirely different approach to these problems, it is a perfect complement to many other approaches Western medical doctors recommend for the following health issues.

Cardiovascular Health

According to Chinese medicine, the heart has special significance in TCM because it's considered to be the "ruler" of all the organs in the body. When you're healthy and everything in your body is balanced, your heart is a caring and good-natured leader. The heart is also especially important in TCM because it is thought to contain the shen, which is loosely translated to mean "soul" or "spirit" but also includes thoughts and feelings (which is why it's sometimes referred to as the heart-mind). Because the heart is so closely connected to emotions in TCM, doing things to keep you mentally healthy—practicing self-awareness, openly expressing yourself, spending time with other people—is often advised as a way of taking care of the heart.

When it comes to preventing heart problems, acupuncture has been shown to be a safe and useful tool. A review paper published in the *Journal of the American College of Cardiology* showed that acupuncture could be useful either alongside or instead of conventional treatment for prevention of heart disease.[4] It is thought that the effect was due to improvement in blood pressure, cholesterol, inflammation, and blood sugar—all risk factors for atherosclerosis, which causes heart attack and stroke. And a study conducted at the University of California, Irvine's Susan Samueli Center for Integrative Medicine found that regular acupuncture treatments can lower hypertension by stimulating the release of an opioid found in the brain stem region that controls blood pressure.[5] Other research suggests acupuncture may improve blood flow to the heart in patients with coronary heart disease.[6] Although I don't recommend acupuncture alone to treat cardiovascular problems, it could be an effective complement, especially since it doesn't interact with any medications.

Tai chi may be an effective recovery technique for people who have experienced heart failure. In one study, a hundred outpatients with systolic heart failure were divided into two groups. One completed a twelve-week tai chi program, while the other, a control group, spent an equivalent amount of time receiving education about their condition. By the end of the twelve weeks, those in the tai chi group had greater improvements in quality of life and mood.[7]

Prostate Health

Prostatitis, as described in Chapter 9, is a common condition, affecting 9 percent of men in the United States. It's the number one urinary tract issue for men under fifty and the third most common one for those who are fifty and up. Symptoms of prostatitis include:

- Pain in the pelvic area, including the lower back and abdomen
- Pain during and/or after urination
- Frequent urination and/or urgency
- Interrupted or weak stream of urine

Western approaches can be frequently unsuccessful in getting rid of symptoms of chronic prostatitis, but acupuncture has been shown to help improve symptoms after twice-weekly treatment for six weeks. Acupuncture is not meant to be a one-time treatment, so for any condition you might be receiving acupuncture, I recommend at least six sessions before deciding whether or not it is helping.

Acupuncture can also work to complement conventional treatment for prostate cancer. Hormone-blockade therapy is often used to reduce the production of testosterone, because the hormone can stimulate prostate cancer cell growth. While suppressing androgens is an effective method for slowing or stopping the growth of cancer, it can cause miserable side effects like hot flashes. Acupuncture has been shown to provide relief from these symptoms in a small study.[8]

JACK: QUITTING SMOKING WITH THE HELP OF ACUPUNCTURE

Some years ago, I worked with a patient named Jack. In most ways, Jack was in phenomenal shape, particularly for a man in his mid-forties. He ran five miles every day, lifted weights, and ate really well. But Jack had a vice he couldn't seem to overcome—he smoked. He'd been doing it since he was in college, and while he had managed to cut back considerably, he still averaged a few cigarettes every day. His habit didn't seem to be slowing him down, but we both knew it was only a matter of time before it started to take a serious toll on his health. Jack had tried several times to quit smoking cold turkey without success, but he wasn't into the idea of nicotine replacement therapy (like the patch) or any other medication. My recommendation as his physician? I sent him to an acupuncturist.

Jack saw the acupuncturist and was given treatment with needles. She also stuck tiny seeds onto a point on his ear with a small piece of medical tape. She told Jack to apply pressure to the seed with his fingers a few times every day between acupuncture sessions. Sure enough, his cravings for cigarettes diminished. He reported that it was as if some outside force had made him lose his taste for smoking. He even lit up a few times, only to put the cigarette out after a few puffs, because it just wasn't as appealing.

Acupuncture can be extremely useful for people who want to quit smoking, especially those looking to do it without medication. When treating smokers, acupuncturists usually focus on specific points in the ears that help suppress the urge to smoke. These points are thought to access cranial nerves, stimulating the nervous system to calm cravings and relieve acute withdrawal symptoms like irritability and fatigue. I also recommend ear seeds—little seeds that the TCM practitioner can attach with flesh-colored tape to continue stimulation of these points that control cravings. Also, since acupuncture is believed to promote the release of feel-good endorphins, part of the help in quitting smoking may be from overall mood and sleep improvement. These acupuncture points have been so effective at curbing cravings and addictions in general that the National Acupuncture Detoxification Association has successfully promoted a specific protocol for the treatment of substance abuse.

Practitioners of TCM also recommend herbs like huang lian, tan shen, and *Ginkgo biloba* for their reported anticancer properties. Because both Western cancer care and Chinese herbal medicine are complex, I usually refer my patients to an acupuncturist or other experienced provider about tailoring the right combination of herbs in coordination with treatment by a Western oncologist. It is important to make sure that herbal treatments don't interfere with chemotherapy or radiation; because these herbs are so powerful, they can have interactions with other treatments just like Western drugs can. Specifically, if a Chinese herbal formulation is a strong antioxidant, it may not be good to use this while getting cancer treatment, such as chemo or radiation, that is meant to kill cancer cells through the process of oxidative damage—you wouldn't want the Chinese herbs protecting the cancer cells. However TCM can be excellent at ameliorating some of the side effects of these toxic but essential therapies.

Sexual Function

Traditional Chinese medicine has many applications in the realm of men's sexual health. Practitioners of TCM have long relied on ginseng to enhance vitality, and Western science supports this use. Research indicates that *Panax ginseng* may improve sexual performance as well as sperm count and quality—meaning it can help with infertility. And other science suggests that ginseng can be used to treat erectile dysfunction (ED). In a study where men who had been clinically diagnosed with ED were given either 900 mg of Korean ginseng a day or a placebo, those who took ginseng experienced significantly better penetration, rigidity, and erection mainte-nance compared to the placebo group.[9]

Acupuncture has also shown promise for treating ED when it's asso-ciated with psychological causes—those not related to injury, side effects of medication, or other physical factors. One study randomly separated twenty-two patients with ED into two groups. The first group received ac-upuncture treatment specific to ED, while the control group was given acupuncture designed to treat headaches. Of the twenty patients who completed the study, around 68 percent of those in the ED treatment group achieved a "satisfactory response," compared to 9 percent of the placebo group.[10]

As has been discussed in Chapter 11, a common (and no less frustrating) problem is premature ejaculation (PE). An estimated one in three men struggles with this issue from time to time. A randomized controlled trial comparing the effects of the antidepressant Paxil (paroxetine), a medi-cation used to treat PE since its primary and very reliable side effect is that it delays orgasm, and acupuncture found that acupuncture had an ejaculation-delaying effect that was not as strong as the medication but was significantly stronger than placebo.[11]

Back Pain

As the number of people addicted to opioids grows to horrifying heights, practitioners and patients alike are searching for ways to manage pain without medication. Acupuncture has such strong evidence behind its use-fulness for pain that in 2017 the American College of Physicians issued guidelines recommending it (along with manual therapy like massage or chiropractic care) as a first step for treating acute or subacute low back pain. Numerous have shown improvements in pain and decreased need for medications for back pain with acupuncture use.

Insomnia and Recovery from Injuries

Acupuncture can help improve relaxation and even boost melatonin produc-tion, the hormone responsible for triggering sleep in our brains. Injury re-covery depends on good sleep and relaxation for healing. Acupuncture has also been shown to help with muscle soreness after aggressive workouts. Another treatment modality within TCM, cupping, involves the use of glass suction cups to help move qi around the body. Cupping is used by athletes to help with recovery, as it helps bring more blood flow to those areas that need repair. That increased blood flow is visible as round red welts that can last for days after cupping. Swimmer Michael Phelps made cupping famous during the 2016 summer Olympics, where he undertook cupping treatments during the course of winning his five gold medals.

The Bottom Line

TCM is a powerful modality that can be used alongside other modalities in prevention or in treatment. Acupuncture, particularly, is an incredible tool because of its accessibility and lack of side effects. As a complementary therapy, it can be used alongside conventional treatment for everything from high blood pressure to infertility, and it may even help you kick a bad habit like smoking. If you're interested in Chinese herbs, be sure to get them from a reliable source and check with your doctor about interactions with any Western medications you are taking.

Notes

1. Berry York et al., "Acupuncture in Military Medicine," in *Acupuncture in Modern Medicine*, edited by Lucy L. Chen and Tsung O. Cheng, 327–346 (Rijeka, Croatia: InTech, 2013), doi: 0.5772/55146, https://cdn.intechopen.com/pdfs-wm/43344.pdf.
2. Nicole Bauke, "Battlefield Acupuncture? Yes, It Exists, and the Military Is Using It to Fight Troops' Pain," *Military Times*, February 10, 2018, https://www.militarytimes.com/news/your-military/2018/02/09/battlefield-acupuncture-yes-it-exists-and-the-military-is-using-it-to-fight-troops-pain.
3. H. Zu et al., "Neural Mechanisms of Acupuncture as Revealed by fMRI Studies," *Autonomic Neuroscience: Basic and Clinical* 190 (2015): 1–9, doi: 10.1016/j.autneu.2015.03.006.
4. Panpan Hao et al., "Traditional Chinese Medicine for Cardiovascular Disease," *Journal of the American College of Cardiology* 69, no. 24 (2017): 2952–2966, doi: 10.1016/j.jacc.2017.04.041.
5. Min Li et al., "Repetitive Electroacupuncture Attenuates Cold-Induced Hypertension Through Enkephalin in the Rostral Ventral Lateral Medulla," *Scientific Reports* 6 (2016), art. 35791, doi: 10.1038/srep35791.
6. "Acupuncture for Coronary Heart Disease Discovery," HealthCMi, December 3, 2013, http://www.healthcmi.com/Acupuncture-Continuing-Education-News/1206-acupuncture-for-coronary-heart-disease-new-discovery.

7. G. Y. Yeh et al., "Tai Chi Exercise in Patients with Chronic Heart Failure: A Randomized Clinical Trial," *Archives of Internal Medicine* 171, no. 8 (2011): 750–757, doi: 10.1001/archinternmed.2011.150.

8. M. Hammar et al., "Acupuncture Treatment of Vasomotor Symptoms in Men with Prostatic Carcinoma: A Pilot Study," *Journal of Urology* 161, no. 3 (1999): 853–856, doi: 10.1016/S0022-5347(01)61789-0.

9. K. W. Leung and A. S. Wong, "Ginseng and Male Reproductive Function," *Spermatogenesis* 3, no. 3 (2013): e26391, doi: 10.4161/spmg.26391.

10. P. E. Engelhardt et al., "Acupuncture in the Treatment of Psychogenic Erectile Dysfunction: First Results of a Prospective Randomized Placebo-Controlled Study," *International Journal of Impotence Research* 15, no. 5 (2003): 343–346, doi: 10.1038/sj.ijir.3901021.

11. D. Sunay et al., "Acupuncture Versus Paroxetine for the Treatment of Premature Ejaculation: A Randomized, Placebo-Controlled Clinical Trial," *European Urology* 59, no. 5 (2011): 765–771, doi: 10.1016/ j.eururo.2011.01.019.

Resources

State laws vary widely in terms of what kind of training, certification, and licensing is required for an individual to perform acupuncture. With that in mind, here are some resources to guide you:

- Acupuncture Now Foundation, https://acupuncturenowfoundation.org/ find-qualified-acupuncturist-usa.
- National Certification Commission for Acupuncture and Oriental Medicine (NCCAOM)
- Acufinder.com Acupuncture Referral Service, https://www.acufinder. com.
- X. Stevenson, T. Shusheng, and C. Yuan, *Handbook of Traditional Chinese Medicine* (Singapore: World Scientific, 2014).
- Michael Tierra, *The Way of Chinese Herbs* (New York: Gallery Books, 1998).

16

Ayurveda for Men

Ayurveda is generally considered to be the oldest system of medicine, originating some five thousand years ago. Loosely translated from the Sanskrit, Ayurveda means "science of life," and it's a holistic healing modality that emphasizes the connection of all things.

While modern medicine in the West tends to focus on eradicating symptoms, Ayurveda is as much about preventing illness as it is about curing it. To this end, aspects of a person's lifestyle, like diet, exercise, and mental fitness, are considered as important for healing as medication. According to the Ayurvedic system, balance is key, and a state of health is achieved when mind, body, and spirit are in harmony. This contrasts sharply with the focus of Western medicine primarily on physical symptoms (or lack thereof) as an indication of health.

Ayurveda holds that there are three different mind-body constitutions, called doshas, that are responsible for guiding our thoughts, feelings, and actions. Each of us has all three doshas within us, but in different combinations and proportions. When our three doshas are balanced, we're in good health. When this balance is disrupted, diseases can begin to develop. Different behaviors—eating too much of a certain food, staying up too late, spending too much time alone, avoiding exercise—aggravate different doshas, leading to an imbalance of the three. We are born with our individual predisposition to be more dominant in one or two doshas, so our health is best when we are able to keep the three in balance. Here are the three doshas:

Vata is made up of air and space elements. A person who is vata-dominant will likely possess some or all of these characteristics:
- Enthusiasm
- Lots of energy
- Creativity
- Willingness and ability to change

A person with an excess or imbalance of vata may struggle with issues like anxiety, insomnia, and restlessness.

Pitta is made up of fire and water elements. A person who is pitta-dominant will likely possess some or all of these characteristics:
- Intelligence
- Intensity
- Drive
- Strong leadership skills

A person with an excess or imbalance of pitta may struggle with issues like irritability, compulsive behavior, and aggression.

Kapha is made up of water and earth elements. A person who is kapha-dominant will likely possess some or all of these characteristic:
- Patience
- Honesty
- Stability
- A desire to care for and nurture others

A person with an excess or imbalance of kapha may struggle with issues like depression, weight gain, and lethargy.

Curious about which of the three doshas dominates your constitution? An Ayurvedic practitioner can help you determine which of these is "your" dosha, or you can use the questionnaire in Table 16.1 to guide you. It asks about your baseline constitution—how you would describe your fundamental nature since you were a child, before any diseases or major life changes affected your nature. Simply check off which is the closest description of yourself from this perspective, then count the number of checks in each column. The column with the most checks would be your predominant dosha.

After you check your dosha type, you can use Table 16.2 to determine how out of balance you might be with respect to your doshas. Remember, the goal in Ayurveda is to maintain a balance of the forces on the mind and body represented by the three doshas. Answer the questions according to how you have been feeling for the last few months.

Table 16.1 Part I of the Dosha Questionnaire

Frame	I am thin, lanky, and slender, with prominent joints and thin muscles.	I have a medium, symmetrical build, with good muscle development.	I have a large, round, or stocky build. My frame is broad, stout, or thick.
Weight	Low; I may forget to eat, or I have a tendency to lose weight.	Moderate; it is easy for me to gain or lose weight if I put my mind to it.	Heavy; I gain weight easily and have difficulty losing it.
Eyes	My eyes are small and active.	I have a penetrating gaze.	I have large, pleasant eyes.
Complexion	My skin is dry, rough, or thin.	My skin is warm, reddish in color, and prone to irritation.	My skin is thick, moist, and smooth.
Hair	My hair is dry, brittle, or frizzy.	My hair is fine with a tendency toward early thinning or graying.	I have abundant, thick, and oily hair.
Joints	My joints are thin and prominent and have a tendency to make cracking sounds.	My joints are loose and flexible.	My joints are large, well knit, and padded.

(*continued*)

Table 16.1 continued

Sleep Pattern	I am a light sleeper with a tendency to awaken easily.	I am a moderately sound sleeper, usually needing less then eight hours to feel rested.	My sleep is deep and long. I tend to awaken slowly in the morning.
Body Temperature	My hands are usually cold and I prefer warm environments.	I am usually warm, regardless of the season, and prefer cooler environments.	I am adaptable to most temperatures but do not like cold, wet days.
Temperament	I am lively and enthusiastic by nature. I like to change.	I am purposeful and intense. I like to convince.	I am easygoing and accepting. I like to support.
Under Stress	I become anxious and/or worried.	I become irritable and/ or aggressive.	I become withdrawn and/or reclusive.
Your Dosha Type (determine by adding up how many you checked for each type)	**Vata Score:**	**Pitta Score:**	**Kapha Score:**

You can look at the numbers to see where you scored high in mind or body. An Ayurvedic practitioner can guide you toward treatments that incorporate suggestions for diet, movement, supplements, and other self-care practices that can help you get things more into balance. This can treat issues as well as prevent future ones.

JEFF, CHEST PAIN HELPED BY AN AYURVEDIC APPROACH

At age forty-six, Jeff was a high achiever who had risen quickly in his job at a large bank. Between work and family obligations, he didn't have much time to exercise, and he usually ate a quick lunch of a sandwich and chips at his desk while he answered emails. While his doctor (whom he saw every couple of years when he got sick with a typical flu or cold) had told him he should have a full checkup, he hadn't gotten around to it. Still, he hadn't had any major health issues—until he awoke around three o'clock one morning with a feeling of chest pressure. He was ready to take an antacid and go back to bed, but his partner called 911 out of concern. When he got to the emergency room, Jeff was shocked to hear he had had a small heart attack. The doctors rushed him to the catheterization lab, where they inserted a stent into the clogged artery around his heart.

He had gone so quickly to the emergency room after feeling pressure in his chest that he hadn't sustained much damage to his heart. But it was a real wake-up call for him: he needed to prevent a bigger, more life-changing (or possibly even life-ending) heart attack or stroke. The problem was, he wasn't sure what he could do besides taking all the medications his cardiologist had started him on. The cardiac rehab program didn't seem rigorous enough to be optimal.

Jeff had seven-year-old twins at home, so he was extremely motivated to do all he needed to get healthier. As a successful and busy businessman, he was used to taking an aggressive approach to problem-solving. He liked the idea that Ayurveda was a complete system, incorporating aspects of mind and body and using many interventions besides just medications to help get him more into balance.

In a long initial appointment, the Ayurvedic doctor asked Jeff about what kind of kid he'd been, about his hobbies and favorite colors, and about how he acted at work and at home, in addition to the standard medical questions. The doctor then explained to Jeff what was happening from an Ayurvedic perspective. Given his natural strong work ethic and overachieving tendencies, the doctor felt Jeff was born with a pitta predisposition, able to be a real leader and to move mountains, but he had been so stressed and so focused on work that his pitta disposition was causing him to be more irritable and to bottle up stress, which in turn was making his heart sick. The doctor recommended mindfulness meditation, a minimum of eight hours of sleep a night, a change in some aspects of what he ate, and several supplements. For example, the doctor suggested that Jeff start each day with warm water and lemon, eat cooling foods, avoid spicy or salty foods, and eat regular meals.

After a few weeks, Jeff felt more relaxed but was still able to stay focused and effective. He could feel that his stress level had declined, and he knew that because he no longer constantly felt on edge, he was lowering his risk of a second, perhaps more serious heart attack.

Table 16.2 Part II of the Dosha Questionnaire

Scale: 1 (not at all), 2 (slightly), 3 (somewhat), 4 (moderately), 5 (very)

1	I've been feeling worried or anxious.	1	2	3	4		5
2	I've been having difficulty falling asleep or have been awakening easily.	1	2	3	4		5
3	I've been feeling restless or uneasy.	1	2	3	4		5
4	I've been acting impulsively or inconsistently.	1	2	3	4		5
5	I've been more forgetful than usual.	1	2	3	4		5

Vata Mind Score: ____

6	My daily schedule of eating meals, going to sleep, or awakening has been inconsistent from day to day	1	2	3	4		5
7	My digestion has been irregular, with gas or bloating	1	2	3	4		5
8	My bowel movements have been hard, dry, or occurring less than once per day.	1	2	3	4		5
9	My skin has been dry or flaky.	1	2	3	4		5
10	I've been having a number of physical concerns.	1	2	3	4		5

Vata Body Score: ____

11	I've been feeling irritable or impatient.	1	2	3	4		5

(continued)

Table 16.2 continued

12	I've been feeling critical and intolerant.	1 2 3 4	5
13	I've been behaving compulsively, with difficulty stopping once I've started a project.	1 2 3 4	5
14	I've been strongly opinionated, freely sharing my point of view without being asked.	1 2 3 4	5
15	I've been feeling frustrated with other people.	1 2 3 4	5

Pitta Mind Score: ___

16	My skin has felt hot and irritable, or has been breaking out easily.	1 2 3 4	5
17	Spicy foods, while I might enjoy them, have not been agreeing with me.	1 2 3 4	5
18	I've been having acid indigestion or heartburn.	1 2 3 4	5
19	I've been feeling overheated, have had a low-grade fever, or have been having hot flashes.	1 2 3 4	5
20	My bowels have been loose or moving more then twice per day.	1 2 3 4	5

Pitta Body Score: ___

21	I've been dealing with conflict by withdrawing.	1 2 3 4	5

Complementary Medicine and Men's Health

Table 16.2 continued

22	I've been accumulating more clutter than usual in my life.	1 2 3 4	5
23	I've been maintaining my routine and feeling resistant to changing my pace.	1 2 3 4	5
24	I've been having difficulty leaving a relationship, job, or situation even though it is no longer nourishing me.	1 2 3 4	5
25	I've been spending more times watching than participating in athletic activity.	1 2 3 4	5

Kapha Mind Score: ____

26	I've been holding on to extra pounds.	1 2 3 4	5
27	I've been having difficulty getting going in the morning.	1 2 3 4	5
28	My digestion has been slow, or I've been feeling heavy after a meal.	1 2 3 4	5
29	I've had sinus congestion or excessive phlegm in my respiratory tract.	1 2 3 4	5
30	I've been feeling drowsy or sluggish after meals.	1 2 3 4	5

Kapha Body Score: ____

Ayurveda for Men

The Main Elements of Ayurveda

Because it's a holistic system of medicine, Ayurveda encompasses a number of different components, but the primary ones are diet, herbal medicine, meditation, and yoga.

Diet

With its emphasis on digestion, Ayurveda revolves around the idea that you are what you eat.

Ayurvedic medicine holds that good digestion is essential for health; when it is compromised, a toxic substance called ama is produced, and illness is given an opportunity to develop.

One of the central tenets of Ayurvedic eating is adherence to both daily and seasonal rhythms. Ayurvedic practitioners generally advise making lunch your largest meal of the day to enhance digestion and boost energy levels, and they suggest modifying your diet seasonally by eating warming foods in the winter, cleansing foods in the spring, and cooling foods in the summer, but specifics may depend on your dosha. Here are some more general suggestions for eating the Ayurvedic way:

- Choose foods according to your dosha.
- Follow a diet that's generally plant-based.
- Focus on colorful, freshly prepared foods.
- Try to incorporate the six tastes into every meal: sweet, sour, salty, bitter, pungent, astringent.
- Try to avoid processed and refined foods.
- Eat slowly and mindfully.
- Don't eat in front of the TV (or any other screen).
- Watch portion size and avoid overindulging.
- Eat primarily cooked foods to aid the digestive process.
- Include healthy oils (in Ayurveda, butter or ghee, which is clarified butter, is considered healthy) with your meal.

Examples of Recommended Foods According to Your Dosha

Dosha needing to be balanced	Vata	Kapha	Pitta
	Sweet, salty, sour foods	Warming foods	Cooling foods
	Berries	Berries	Watermelon
	Avocados	Black beans	Celery
	Sweet potatoes	Pumpkin seeds	Apples
	Pistachios	Peppers	Coconut
	Lentils	Cherries	Cabbage
	Beets	Lemons, limes	Kale
	Peaches	Spinach	Pasta

Herbal Medicine

The history of herbalism in Ayurveda is rich, and many herbs that were once considered purely Ayurvedic have gained popularity in the West. Following are descriptions of just some of the many plants used. As with any supplement, you should look for reputable manufacturers of quality Ayurvedic herbal products, preferably with the help of an experienced practitioner. I also recommend checking with your doctor before starting a new medicine to avoid interactions or other problems.

Ashwagandha

This herb has become increasingly popular in contemporary medicine. We covered this in Chapter 4 in the description of adaptogens, herbs that can help your body adapt to whatever difficult circumstances it's facing. They work to provide balance in your system. Feeling anxious? Adaptogens help calm you. Tired? They help energize you. They can even do both at the same time! Regardless of which way you're swinging, adaptogens can bring you back to the center, all without disrupting normal biological function. They increase our ability to cope with and respond to whatever comes our way. Given the hectic pace of twenty-first-century life, you can understand why so many people are turning to these powerful herbs.

Adaptogens like ashwagandha are especially respected for their unique ability to help the body handle stress and to even lower the stress hormone cortisol. In a study looking at the effect of ashwagandha on individuals with a history of chronic stress, those who took ashwagandha capsules twice a day for sixty days had their stress and cortisol levels significantly lowered compared to a placebo group.[1]

Side effects to consider with Ashwagandha include slight lowering of blood sugar and blood pressure, so if you are prone to hypoglycemia or light-headedness upon standing, be careful with this herb. There is some concern that it can increase immune function, even in those with autoimmune diseases, situations where an increase in immune system function would not be favorable.

Boswellia

Also known as Indian frankincense, this resin has played a role in medicine and spirituality since ancient times. Long relied upon by Ayurvedic practitioners to treat conditions like arthritis and respiratory illness, boswellia has gained the attention of modern scientists thanks to one of its compounds, boswellic acid. Research indicates boswellic acid possess powerful anti-inflammatory properties that may help treat autoimmune conditions like rheumatoid arthritis, Crohn's disease, and ulcerative colitis.[2] Its ability to fight inflammation means boswellic acid could be useful for relieving joint pain and other aches as well. I frequently recommend a product that combines boswellia with quercetin and curcumin (discussed later) as a natural pain reliever and anti-inflammatory, sort of like a natural Motrin (ibuprofen).

The effects of boswellia on the skin have also been examined, with remarkable results. In one study, fifteen volunteers applied a cream containing 0.5 percent boswellic acids to one side of their faces while using the same cream minus the boswellic acids on the other side for 30 days. At the end of the study, the facial skin treated with the boswellic acids cream showed significant improvements in roughness and fine lines as well as increased elasticity—all without any adverse reactions.[3]

Triphala

This popular Ayurvedic remedy is actually a combination of three fruits: amla, bibhitaki, and haritaki. Triphala facilitates healthy digestion, which is absolutely necessary for overall health according to Ayurveda. This detoxifying formula is frequently recommended for constipation, bloating, and other gastrointestinal issues. I have found it to be one of the most effective natural treatments for constipation, but it doesn't work with just one dose, like a traditional laxative. You need to take it daily for a week or so to make your bowel movements more regular.

Based on research, triphala also seems to have anticancer effects. A 2015 study looking at the effects of triphala on colon cancer cells and human colon cancer stem cells found the remedy was able to both suppress the spread of and cause the death of colon cancer stem cells, indicating its anticancer potential.[4] As I discuss in the section of this chapter on prostate health, triphala may also be helpful for treating prostate cancer.

Turmeric

If you've paid even the slightest bit of attention to the world of wellness lately, you've likely heard some buzz about turmeric. Derived from the underground stems (rhizomes) of the plant *Curcuma longa*, which is a member of the ginger family, turmeric is considered by some to be most valuable Ayurvedic herb. Traditionally, practitioners of Ayurveda have used turmeric to treat conditions affecting the respiratory system and liver (among many other things), and modern science supports the use of turmeric to treat an astounding array of health issues through its potent anti-inflammatory effects. Some of these include:

- *Arthritis.* In an Italian study of patients with osteoarthritis in one or both knees, those who took a turmeric formulation for ninety days showed a 58 percent reduction in overall pain and stiffness compared to controls.

They were also able to reduce their need for painkillers like aspirin and ibuprofen by 63 percent compared to patients on conventional medical therapy alone.[5]

- *Inflammatory bowel disease.* The active compound in turmeric, curcumin, has been shown to relieve the symptoms of IBD. A data review looking at studies of curcumin for IBD found it has potential as an adjunct therapy as well as on its own.[6]
- *Depression or other mood disorders.* A study where fifty-six patients with major depressive disorder took either curcumin or placebo capsules for eight weeks found those who took curcumin showed significant improvement compared to the placebo group.[7]

Turmeric is limited by low bioavailability, meaning a relatively small amount enters your body's circulation, but the absorption can be improved dramatically when taken with black pepper, so the better turmeric supplements will have pepper (or piperine, one of the substances in black pepper) added. There are also liposomal preparations that are very well absorbed.

Meditation

An important component of the Ayurvedic treatment plan for Jeff, whom I introduced earlier in this chapter, was meditation. In his case, he was benefiting from mindfulness-style meditation. But sometimes Ayurvedic practitioners will recommend more of a traditional mantra-style meditation.

The benefits of meditation have been borne out by numerous studies, as noted in Chapter 6. One study from Harvard Medical School showed that people with generalized anxiety who followed a stress reduction program based on meditation were considerably less anxious than those in a control group who were taught other stress management techniques.[8]

Some Ayurvedic practitioners believe sunrise and sunset are ideal for meditation, but there's really not a bad time to reap the benefits of this calming practice. There are plenty of smartphone apps that will teach you how to meditate if you're so inclined. Check out Chapter 6 for specific resources.

Yoga

This practice has become so popular in America that its association with Ayurvedic medicine is sometimes forgotten. According to *The Complete Illustrated Guide to Ayurveda*, the word *yoga* comes from the Sanskrit *yuga*, "to unite" or "to join," and it is designed to bring harmony through the mastery of the mind as well as the body. Originating in India several thousand years ago, yoga continues to be a pillar of Ayurveda. Although focus in the West tends to be on poses, yoga is actually multifaceted. Two of the main components of Ayurvedic yoga practice are asanas and pranayama. Asanas are the various poses you perform during your yoga practice. Done correctly, they can bring about a state of deep calm while helping your body function optimally. Pranayama is a method of deep, controlled breathing from the diaphragm. Awareness of one's breath is an integral part of yoga and meditation.

Yoga can provide a number of physical and spiritual benefits, including relief of one of the most common problems encountered by men, back pain. In a randomized controlled trial including over three hundred people with chronic or recurrent low back pain, participants were assigned to either usual care or a twelve-class yoga program that lasted three months. Based on questionnaires filled out by study participants, researchers concluded that subjects who participated in in the yoga program experienced greater improvements in back function than those who received usual care.[9] Other studies have also shown improvements in pain, reduction in the amount of medication needed for back pain, and even a drop in depression scores among people who use yoga for back pain. I have seen over and over again the power of a regular yoga practice to really help my patients with chronic back pain.

The Benefits of Ayurveda Specifically in Men's Health

Having scratched the surface of this complex healing modality, let's turn to the role of Ayurveda in men's health. As we examine its application to various conditions, bear in mind that Ayurvedic medicine focuses on addressing the underlying cause of illness instead of specific symptoms. As such, a personalized treatment plan devised by an Ayurvedic practitioner will typically include advice on diet, exercise, and self-awareness as well as herbal medicine.

Cardiovascular Health

The focus of Ayurveda on preventing disease by promoting a healthy lifestyle is important for protecting the heart. Study after study has shown how important physical movement is for keeping the cardiovascular system strong. What you eat, too, is key for heart health in Ayurveda, which emphasizes the use of food as medicine and typically favors a plant-based diet.

Guggul, an herb that features prominently in Ayurvedic medicine, has demonstrated potential for improving heart health. Research suggests that one bioactive constituent of guggul, called guggulsterone, possesses lipid-lowering, antioxidant, and anti-inflammatory properties.[10] Other studies on the ability of guggul to lower cholesterol have yielded mixed results, but guggul could be an option for patients with very mildly elevated cholesterol levels when used under the advice of a doctor and an Ayurvedic practitioner.

Another Ayurvedic herb called bitter melon could reduce cardiovascular risk factors, particularly for men with diabetes or prediabetes. Bitter melon may help regulate blood sugar, and animal studies show it can lower triglyceride levels as well.[11]

Prostate Health

Ayurvedic medicine may offer some relief for those men dealing with the very common condition benign prostatic hyperplasia (BPH). As discussed in Chapter 9, BPH is characterized by frequent urination, intermittent or interrupted urine stream, an urgent need to urinate, and nocturia (waking at night to urinate). The herb tribulus has long been used in Ayurveda for urinary problems, and a study found the diuretic and contractile effects of tribulus may even help passage of urinary stones.[12] Other Ayurvedic herbal medicines have also traditionally been used to alleviate symptoms associated with BPH, depending on your own specific constitution. A trained practitioner can help identify what would be best for you.

For prostate cancer, the herbal formulation triphala may be beneficial, due to a bioactive constituent known as gallic acid. In a study looking at its effect on prostate cancer cells, gallic acid was found to have promising anticancer activity.[13]

Cancer Prevention

When it comes to preventing cancer and other chronic illness, Ayurveda has the same principle as many other healing modalities: balance. Taking time to care for yourself—both body and mind—by eating well, exercising, meditating, managing stress, and getting enough rest is what an Ayurvedic practitioner would likely recommend if you asked about disease prevention.

As far as specific Ayurvedic herbs for cancer, as I said, turmeric has the potential to treat many different health conditions. In 2005, researchers from the University of Texas M. D. Anderson Cancer Center found that curcumin (the anti-inflammatory compound in turmeric) blocks a key biological pathway needed for development of melanoma and other cancers. Other studies support turmeric's anticancer potential, focusing on its ability to suppress the growth of tumor cells.[14]

Sexual Function

As previously mentioned, we sometimes use an SSRI medication to help with premature ejaculation (PE). I talked in Chapter 15 about how acupuncture can be a drug-free treatment option, and research suggests yoga may help as well. A study comparing the effects of yoga and Prozac (fluoxetine) on PE divided participants into two groups, with thirty-eight people doing yoga and thirty people taking medication. At the end of the study period, all thirty-eight people in the yoga group showed statistically significant improvement in PE, compared to twenty-five out of thirty (around 82 percent) of the SSRI group.[15]

The Ayurvedic herb ashwagandha has traditionally been considered an aphrodisiac, which isn't surprising when you think about how often psychological factors like stress and anxiety—conditions that adaptogens such as ashwagandha excel at moderating—can dampen libido. Ashwagandha has also been shown to improve infertility. In a pilot study where men with low sperm count were randomly given either ashwagandha extract or a placebo for ninety days, the ashwagandha group experienced a 167 percent increase in sperm count, a 53 percent increase in semen volume, and a 57 percent increase in sperm motility compared to the placebo group.[16]

Ayurveda in Prevention

While I've included some tips for Ayurvedic treatment of some conditions of greatest concern to men, the value of this type of medicine really lies in its focus on prevention. Ayurveda teaches that the seeds of disease are present long before physical manifestations develop. The extensive inquiry that an Ayurvedic specialist conducts is meant to identify imbalances that can lead to disease years later if not addressed now by eliminating dosha imbalances.

The Bottom Line

As a physician who advocates lifestyle changes to help my patients prevent illness and achieve their goals, I'm a big fan of Ayurveda's holistic approach. Since there's much more to this ancient modality than I can cover in a single chapter, I suggest working with a practitioner who can tailor a treatment just for you.

Notes

1. K. Chandrasekhar et al., "A Prospective, Randomized Double-Blind, Placebo-Controlled Study of Safety and Efficacy of a High-Concentration Full-Spectrum Extract of Ashwagandha Root in Reducing Stress and Anxiety in Adults," *Indian Journal of Psychological Medicine* 34, no. 3 (2012): 255, doi:10.4103/0253-7176.106022.
2. H. P. T. Ammon, "Boswellic Acids and Their Role in Chronic Inflammatory Diseases," in *Anti-Inflammatory Nutraceuticals and Chronic Diseases*, edited by S. C. Gupta, S. Prasad, and B. B. Aggarwal, 291–327 (Cham, Switzerland: Springer, 2016), doi: 10.1007/978-3-319-41334-1_13.
3. Alessandra Pedretti et al., "Effects of Topical Boswellic Acid on Photo and Age-Damaged Skin: Clinical, Biophysical, and Echographic Evaluations in a Double-Blind, Randomized, Split-Face Study," *Planta Medica* 76, no. 6 (2009): 555–560, doi: 10.1055/s-0029-1240581.
4. Ramakrishna Vadde et al., "Triphala Extract Suppresses Proliferation and Induces Apoptosis in Human Colon Cancer Stem Cells via Suppressing c-Myc/Cyclin D1 and Elevation of Bax/Bcl-2 Ratio," *BioMed Research International*, 2015, art. ID 649263, doi: 10.1155/2015/649263.
5. G. Belcaro et al., "Product-Evaluation Registry of Meriva®, Curcumin-Phosphatidylcholine Complex, for the Complementary Management of Osteoarthritis." *Panminerva Medica* 52, no. 2 supp. 1 (2010): 55–62.
6. R. A. Taylor and M. C. Leonard, "Curcumin for Inflammatory Bowel Disease: A Review of Human Studies," *Alternative Medicine Review* 16, no. 2 (2011): 153–156.
7. A. L. Lopresti et al., "Curcumin for the Treatment of Major Depression: A Randomised, Double-Blind, Placebo Controlled Study," *Journal of Affective Disorders* 167 (2014): 368–375, doi: 10.1016/j.jad.2014.06.001.

8. Elizabeth A. Hoge et al., "Randomized Controlled Trial of Mindfulness Meditation for Generalized Anxiety Disorder," *Journal of Clinical Psychiatry* 74, no. 8 (2013): 786–792, doi: 10.4088/jcp.12m08083.

9. H. E. Tilbrook et al., "Yoga for Chronic Low Back Pain: A Randomized Trial," *Annals of Internal Medicine* 155, no. 9 (2011): 569–578, doi: 10.7326/0003-4819-155-9-201111010-00003.

10. Ruitang Deng, "Therapeutic Effects of Guggul and Its Constituent Guggulsterone: Cardiovascular Benefits," *Cardiovascular Drug Reviews* 25, no. 4 (2007): 375–390, doi:10.1111/j.1527-3466.2007.00023.x.

11. E. Basch, S. Gabardi, and C. Ulbricht, "Bitter Melon (*Momordica charantia*): A Review of Efficacy and Safety," *American Journal of Health-System Pharmacy* 60, no. 4 (2003): 336–359, doi: 10.1093/ajhp/60.4.356.

12. Muneer Al-Ali et al., "*Tribulus terrestris*: Preliminary Study of Its Diuretic and Contractile Effects and Comparison with *Zea mays*," *Journal of Ethnopharmacology* 85, nos. 2–3 (2003): 257–260, doi: 10.1016/s0378-8741(03)00014-x.

13. Larry H. Russell Jr. et al., "Differential Cytotoxicity of Triphala and Its Phenolic Constituent Gallic Acid on Human Prostate Cancer LNCap and Normal Cells," *Anticancer Research* 31, no. 11 (2011): 3739–3745.

14. University of Texas M. D. Anderson Cancer Center, "Potent Spice Works to Block Growth of Melanoma in Lab Test," ScienceDaily, July 14, 2005, www.sciencedaily.com/releases/2005/07/050712232338.htm.

15. V. Dhikav et al., "Yoga in Premature Ejaculation: A Comparative Trial with Fluoxetine," *Journal of Sexual Medicine* 4, no. 6 (2015): 1726–1732, doi: 10.1111/j.1743-6109.2007.00603.x.

16. Vijay R. Ambiye et al., "Clinical Evaluation of the Spermatogenic Activity of the Root Extract of Ashwagandha (*Withania somnifera*) in Oligospermic Males: A Pilot Study," *Evidence-Based Complementary and Alternative Medicine*, 2013, art. ID 571420, doi: 10.1155/2013/571420.

Resources

To connect with a practitioner in your area, see the website of the National Ayurvedic Medical Association (NAMA), http://www.ayurvedanama.org/search/custom.asp?id=945. No states license Ayurvedic practitioners, but this organization certifies practitioners.

One of the most famous Ayurvedic doctors is Deepak Chopra. He has helped to substantially popularize meditation and yoga. The Chopra Center offers many programs, from personal evaluations and

Ayurveda for Men

treatments to actual trainings in Ayurveda; for an introduction to Ayurveda, see https://chopra.com/articles/what-is-ayurveda. His book *Perfect Health* (New York: Three Rivers Press, 2000) is an excellent resource on mind-body health and is rooted in Ayurveda.

For an excellent resource on Ayurvedic herbs, see D. Frawley and V. Lad, *The Yoga of Herbs: An Ayurvedic Guide to Herbal Medicine*, 2nd ed. (Twin Lakes, WI: Lotus Press, 2001).

17

Homeopathy for Men

The system of homeopathic medicine was created in the late 1700s by a German doctor named Samuel Christian Hahnemann. Much like other healing modalities, homeopathy is based on the belief that a state of health is achieved when the mind and the body are balanced, and that this equilibrium is controlled by a "vital force" that works to manage the body's power to heal itself. We understand this largely as a form of energy medicine.

When he established his new system of healing, Dr. Hahnemann chose the name homeopathy from the Greek *homeo*, meaning "similar," and *pathos*, meaning "suffering." This name gets at a guiding principle of homeopathy called the law of similars. More commonly referred to as "like cures like," this means the substances that cause a healthy body to experience certain symptoms can be used to treat similar symptoms in a sick person. An example is the botanical belladonna being used for scarlet fever, since the symptoms of this illness are much like those caused by belladonna poisoning.

The doses used in homeopathy are orders of magnitude less than those used in traditional western medicine. Often homeopathy is taken as tiny round pellets, maybe ten or so at a time, and placed under the tongue. You may have seen one of the most commonly used homeopathic remedies for colds and flu, called Oscillococcinum, which is available at most drugstores.

This medicine is designed to relieve symptoms like body aches, chills, and fatigue.

The doses are so tiny that the effect of homeopathic remedies cannot possibly be from conventional medical pharmacological effects, which depends on chemistry. Instead, homeopathy relies on energy. So while a homeopathic remedy may be in the form of pills, drops, or creams, these forms are merely vehicles for delivering energy. In this way, homeopathic remedies are actually drug-free in that they don't contain the chemical ingredients that make up conventional medicines. This may be why homeopathic remedies are so safe—there has never been a documented incident of toxicity from them. In terms of governmental regulation, the Food and Drug Administration (FDA) hasn't evaluated any product labeled as homeopathic for safety or effectiveness. But that doesn't mean they're not safe. Since homeopathic remedies rely on energy to work and are made from a minuscule amount of active ingredient, they're quite benign.

When people talk about the potency of a homeopathic remedy, they're referring to the concentration of the raw substance that is in the remedy. This impacts the level of energy contained in the medicine. A common way of measuring and labeling this energy is with the centesimal (c) scale. To make a 1c dilution, a homeopath adds one drop of the raw substance, called the mother tincture, to 99 drops of alcohol and shakes vigorously. A 2c is made when a drop of 1c is added to 99 drops of alcohol, and so on.

- 6c is the potency typically indicated for minor physical complaints
- 30c is a medium potency that can help with acute problems because it can affect the psyche while also addressing physical symptoms
- 200c is a fast-acting potency frequently used by practitioners in acute situations with conditions like a high fever or a nasty stomach bug.[1]

It requires a significant amount of training to know what the appropriate homeopathic remedy is for a particular condition. There is no state that licenses homeopaths who aren't either medical doctors (MDs) or naturopathic doctors (NDs) already, but there is certification available for those who are fully trained to testify to their competence. I suggest looking for a practitioner who has been certified in this way or seeking out an ND who practices homeopathy. Often, the practitioner will try to identify one—and only one—particular remedy given the patient's particular symptoms as well as his overall history and general constitution. Practitioners will often spend an hour or more during an initial assessment to come up with the recommended specific remedy.

Just like with supplements, quality can certainly vary from product to product, but there are many trustworthy homeopathic companies out there. For example, Boiron, one of the biggest suppliers of homeopathic medicines in the country, assures consumers that its remedies are manufactured in accordance with the Homeopathic Pharmacopoeia of the United States (HPUS). As long as you work with a professional who's familiar with homeopathic remedies, you will be guided to reputable remedies.

The Homeopathic Essential Remedies

Here are some commonly used single homeopathic remedies. Kept in your medicine cabinet or first-aid kit at home, these can be helpful for treating acute but non-life-threatening symptoms.[2]

Apis: This remedy is said to relieve the pain and swelling from bee stings.

Arnica montana: By far the most well-known homeopathic remedy, Arnica is used to treat bruises, muscle soreness, and other symptoms associated with traumatic injuries. It also helps minimize swelling after surgery.

Belladonna: Among many other things, this remedy can be used to soothe sunstroke.

Calendula: Typically used in gel, cream, or ointment form, this remedy can be used to promote gentle healing of cuts, scrapes, and other skin irritations.

Cantharis: This is a good one for your-first aid kit because it can be used for two common (and painful) types of blisters, those caused by burns and those resulting from friction.

Hypericum: Homeopathic practitioners often recommend this remedy for nerve pain, including toothaches and other dental discomfort.

Ignatia: This remedy is meant to treat mental symptoms rather than physical ones—practitioners often use it to treat acute grief, anxiety, and depression.

Ledum: Keep this one in your first-aid kit and use it to treat puncture wounds and cuts in addition to using topical antibacterial ointments and seeking medical care if warranted.

Nux vomica: Whether you had one too many drinks at the bar or overindulged on ice cream, this remedy may be able to alleviate your discomfort.

Rhus toxicodendron (Rhus tox): This remedy is often indicated for skin and joint disorders. It can be used to ease symptoms of conditions ranging from chicken pox and eczema to arthritic pain and sciatica.

These remedies all look like the same—tiny white pellets. Because they're so diluted and rely on energy medicine, each remedy can be delivered in an identical form. Unlike most oral medications, which are swallowed, homeopathic pellets are meant to be taken sublingually (dissolved under the tongue). On its website, Boiron offers some additional tips for ensuring optimal absorption when you take a homeopathic remedy. Here are some of the suggestions:

- Take medicines in a mouth free of strong flavors like coffee or mint. (For example, don't take your remedy alongside your morning cup of joe.)
- You don't have to worry about whether you should take your remedy with or without food, but you should do it fifteen minutes before or after eating, drinking, or brushing your teeth (especially if you use a minty toothpaste).
- Try to touch the pellets as little as possible to avoid getting moisture and oils from your fingers on them. These substances can coat the pellets and interfere with absorption.

In addition to these individual homeopathic remedies, a handful of commercially prepared homeopathic formulations including a combination of ingredients have found mainstream success thanks to their reputation for efficacy.

T-Relief: Formerly known as Traumeel, this recently reformulated homeopathic analgesic is available in a variety of forms for topical and internal use. Featuring arnica as well as 12 other homeopathics, T-Relief can be used to ease joint, back, and muscle pain. Published studies have shown it to be as effective as oral anti-inflammatory medications for reducing symptoms of inflammation, improving mobility and accelerating recovery from musculoskeletal injuries.[3]

Hyland's Calms Forté: For people who struggle with insomnia—particularly the kind caused by anxiety—but don't want to take a sleeping pill that will make them feel groggy the next day, this can be a gentle yet reportedly effective option.

Similasan eye drops: This beloved brand was founded in Switzerland nearly 40 years ago. Created using traditional homeopathic standards, these various formulas can address concerns like "allergy eyes" and eye strain caused by staring at a computer screen for too long.

Iberogast: This combination of 9 homeopathic remedies is amazing for treating indigestion and gastrointestinal reflux.

Who Can Benefit from Homeopathy?

Homeopathy is a system of healing that relies on energy to balance the body and mind. Men experiencing the following conditions may find homeopathy helpful when used as a complement to conventional treatment:

- High blood pressure[4]
- Heart failure
- Stroke
- Benign prostatic hypertrophy (BPH)
- Infertility
- Sports injuries or trauma
- Arthritis
- Allergies

The Benefits of Homeopathy Specifically in Men's Health

There are specific conditions in men's health that homeopathy can help with. It's important to note that homeopaths seek to match remedies to the patient instead of to the ailment, so different people with the same condition could benefit from very different remedies.

Cardiovascular Health

As is the case with acupuncture, homeopathy is often most effective as a complementary therapy used alongside other treatments. In one study, patients with mild cardiac insufficiency were given either a homeopathic preparation called Cralonin or conventional medication (ACE inhibitors and diuretics). Evaluating treatment efficacy based on fifteen variables, researchers found Cralonin was "non-inferior" to drug therapy (meaning it worked just as well) on all parameters except blood pressure reduction.[5] I do not recommend treating heart failure with homeopathy alone, but science indicates its complementary potential.

Homeopathy may also play a complementary role in stroke recovery. The following remedies are mentioned in the *Encyclopedia of Homeopathy*:

- Arnica montana for a hemorrhagic stroke
- Hyoscyamus for a paralytic stroke
- Opium for a major stroke

Prostate Health

Benign prostatic hypertrophy (BPH) is a common issue among older men, as discussed in Chapter 9. If you are having symptoms from BPH, you may want to consider adding homeopathy to whatever treatment your physician recommends. According to the *Encyclopedia of Homeopathy*, the following can also be helpful for enlarged prostate:

- Apis for urinary retention
- Sabal if urination is difficult
- Baryata carb for frequent urge to urinate and/or a slow urine stream

Since homeopathy treats individuals rather than conditions, I suggest working directly with a trained homeopath to find the right remedy for you. (After you see a doctor, of course.)

Cancer Prevention

In terms of treating cancer, homeopathy alone will never be an appropriate choice, but it may help as a complementary therapy. In one study a hundred rats were injected with cancerous prostate tumor cells and then exposed to five homeopathic remedies for five weeks. At the end of the study period, researchers concluded that the remedies significantly slowed the progression of cancer.[6] Again, such treatment should only be taken in addition to standard Western treatment and under the guidance of an expert.

Conditions like erectile dysfunction can be difficult to treat because they're often caused by a complicated combination of psychological factors like stress, anxiety, and relationship issues. This complexity makes sexual dysfunction an excellent topic of discussion with a homeopath. Since homeopathy focuses on treating an individual's symptoms, it may be worth consulting a homeopathic specialist for the creation of a highly specific treatment plan.

Some studies indicate homeopathy might be helpful for improving male fertility. In one of these studies, forty-five subfertile men were treated with single homeopathic remedies prescribed according to subjects' symptoms for an average of around ten months. Researchers noted significant improvement in sperm density and motility as well as a bump in general patient health.[7] These gains are comparable to those achieved with conventional treatment, so homeopathy could be a good option for men looking to boost their fertility.

Five years ago, I treated a patient named Rick. Rick is an avid cyclist who came to me because he knew I was also an athlete. Rick had been involved in a nasty bike accident while racing, and he was pretty beat up. He had no serious injuries, but lots of bruises and some serious "road rash." Because he was already taking a few prescriptions and didn't want to worry about drug interactions, Rick preferred to avoid painkillers and other conventional medication, and he was wondering if I could recommend an alternative. After a bit of thought, I suggested arnica.

As previously explained, arnica montana is renowned for its ability to heal symptoms like swelling, bruising, and pain related to traumatic injuries. Rick accepted my advice and headed to the nearest health food store to pick some up. A few days later, I got a call from an amazed, grateful, and rapidly healing patient! Rick told me his swelling had gone down considerably and his bruises were less angry-looking after consistent use of oral arnica. He later

Homeopathy for Men

shared his experience with his fellow cyclists, many of whom started carrying arnica in their race kits (which is ideal, since arnica seems to work best for injuries soon after they happen). Since then, I've recommended both oral and topical forms of arnica to countless patients, athletes, and friends, and science supports my anecdotal experience.

Arthritis

Topical homeopathic preparations—especially those featuring arnica—really shine when it comes to treating symptoms of arthritis. (I should clarify that, while they're primarily homeopathic, arnica creams and gels do contain a bit of plant material, so they could also be considered herbal products.) An uncontrolled trial including seventy-nine people with mild to moderate osteoarthritis of the knee found that topical arnica gel produced significant improvements in pain, stiffness, and other measures at both the three- and six-week marks. Only one patient reported an adverse reaction, with 87 percent of participants rating the tolerability of the gel as "good" or "fairly good" and 76 percent saying they'd use it again.[8]

Another randomized, double-blind study comparing the effects of arnica gel and ibuprofen gel for treatment of hand osteoarthritis found no difference between the two groups in pain intensity, hand function, or any other measures, leading researchers to conclude that arnica is "not inferior" to ibuprofen for treating osteoarthritis in the hands.[9] This study may be of special interest to those who wish to avoid the side effects associated with non-steroidal anti-inflammatory drugs (NSAIDs) like ibuprofen.

The Bottom Line

Homeopathy is a complex and fascinating healing modality that may serve to complement conventional treatments for many different conditions. In my practice, I like to mention homeopathic remedies to my patients who are on a lot of different medications because I know I won't need to worry about drug interactions. The concepts behind homeopathy can be difficult to grasp, and I wouldn't begrudge you a healthy amount of skepticism about the whole "energy medicine" thing. But if you approach it with an open mind, you might be surprised by the ways homeopathy enhances your health.

Notes

1. Andrew Lockie, *Encyclopedia of Homeopathy* (London: DK, 2006). This is one of the best resources for information on specific homeopathic remedies.
2. C. Griffith, *The Practical Handbook of Homeopathy* (London: Watkins, 2006).
3. C. Schneider, "Traumeel: An Emerging Option to NSAIDS in the Management of Acute Musculoskeletal Injuries," International Journal of General Medicine 25, no. 4 (2011): 225–234, doi: 10.2147/IJGM.S16709.
4. G. Hitzenberger et al., [Controlled randomized double-blind study for the comparison of the treatment of patients with essential hypertension with homeopathic and with pharmacologically effective drugs], *Wiener klinische Wochenschrift* 94, no. 24 (1982): 665–670.
5. D. Schröder et al., "Efficacy of a Homeopathic Crataegus Preparation Compared with Usual Therapy for Mild (NYHA II) Cardiac Insufficiency: Results of an Observational Cohort Study," *European Journal of Heart Failure* 5, no. 3 (2003): 319–326, doi: 10.1016/s1388-9842(02)00237-4.
6. Wayne B. Jonas et al., "Can Homeopathic Treatment Slow Prostate Cancer Growth?," *Integrative Cancer Therapies* 5, no. 4 (2006): 343–349, doi: 10.1177/1534735406294225.
7. I. Gerhard and E. Wallis, "Individualized Homeopathic Therapy for Male Infertility," *Homeopathy* 91, no. 3 (2002): 133–144, doi: 10.1054/homp.2002.0024.
8. Otto Knuesel et al., "Arnica Montana Gel in Osteoarthritis of the Knee: An Open, Multicenter Clinical Trial," *Advances in Therapy* 19, no. 5 (2002): 209–218, doi: 10.1007/bf02850361.
9. Reto Widrig et al., "Choosing Between NSAID and Arnica for Topical Treatment of Hand Osteoarthritis in a Randomised, Double-Blind Study," *Rheumatology International* 27, no. 6 (2007): 585–591, doi: 10.1007/s00296-007-0304-y.

Resources

You may have noticed how often I mentioned the *Encyclopedia of Homeopathy* by Andrew Lockie, MD, MRCGP, FFHom, in this chapter. That's because I think it's an excellent, easy-to-navigate reference for people interested in learning about homeopathy. It shouldn't replace consultation with a qualified homeopathic practitioner (which in turn isn't an appropriate substitution for seeing a doctor in most cases). Still, it's a good book to have on hand. Here are some other resources for information on homeopathy and/or finding a licensed homeopath in your area. Keep in mind that, as with practitioners of traditional Chinese medicine, licensing rules and regulations for practicing homeopathy vary from state to state.

National Center for Homeopathy (NCH), http://www.homeopathycenter.org/find-homeopath. This site features a practitioner directory made up of professional members of the NCH.

Boiron Homeopathic Medicine Finder, https://www.boironusa.com/mf. Run by the manufacturer of Oscillococcinum and many other remedies, this site allows users to search by symptom(s).

North American Society of Homeopaths (NASH), https://homeopathy.org. This is a membership organization for professional homeopaths, students, schools and homeopathy supporters.

American Institute of Homeopathy (AIH), http://homeopathyusa.org/member-directory.html. This site lets you look for licensed homeopathic practitioners in your state (meaning licensed as MDs or NDs and also trained in homeopathy).

SECTION 4

Conclusion

18

The Future of
Men's Health

have shared many patient stories throughout this book. They all show
elements of approaches to optimal men's health that I have found successful. Now I'd like to share my vision of where I believe we can go in
terms of optimizing the health of men, if we want to truly take advantage of
modern technology and utilize a sophisticated understanding of preventive
medicine tools.

Austin: A Case Study

Austin, who is forty-two, comes in to see me for an optimal health check-in.
He works for a technology corporation, mostly remotely. He's been noticing
he doesn't bounce back as well as he used to after a night out with his
friends, and he is starting to develop a belly, which his partner pointed out.
He hasn't been exercising as much because of his work schedule. It's great
to work from home (or coffee shops), but it also means he never really
gets to clock out and leave work behind. His other concern is that he gets
tired and has a hard time maintaining mental focus every day, usually in

the afternoon. That's when he relies on coffee or energy drinks to give him a boost.

Austin follows whatever diets his friends are talking about and takes supplements according to what he reads in magazines or sees at the pharmacy. He wants to know what the best diet for him really is, what supplements he should take, and what sort of exercise is best for him in order to stay fit. He has some family history of heart disease, so he'd like to make sure he is doing what he can to avoid such problems.

We start by discussing Austin's personal and family medical history. Then we talk about his goals—not his health goals, but what really matters to him. What does he want his heath *for*? He says his goal is to get his own tech start-up going and then cash out, selling the company for a lot of money, before he turns forty-five.

When he scheduled his appointment, we sent him a kit with a swab for him to collect his DNA by brushing the inside of his cheek, so at this initial appointment we have the results of his genetic tests to review. Based on this genetic test, we know he has a few risks for health problems that could waylay his plans. For example, he has one copy of ApoE4, which, as you remember from Chapter 8, increases his risk for heart disease and early Alzheimer's. He also has variations in genes important in detoxification, so he could develop autoimmune problems or fatigue issues if he is not careful to minimize exposure to toxins and make sure to incorporate foods containing compounds that help with detoxification (especially cruciferous vegetables).

His health history and genetic tests inform what other testing we need to do to get a strong sense of Austin's current state of health and individualized health risks. We may want to drill down into his risk for heart disease or his vitamin levels. We may want to investigate his hormones or the levels of heavy metals in his body.[1]

Based on his test results, when Austin comes back in two weeks, I present him with the following plan:

Diet

- Emphasize a low-fat diet with 55 percent of calories from carbohydrates, 25 percent of calories from proteins, and 20 percent of calories from healthy fats (in accordance with his specific genetic makeup).
- Decrease sugar and white bread, white pasta, and white potatoes for .optimal weight.

- Eat foods rich in natural folic acid (greens, chickpeas and beans, asparagus, broccoli, avocado) to help his body detoxify, given his genetic profile.
- Limit added sugars, juices, and soda.
- Eat broccoli sprouts when possible to help with detoxification.
- Emphasize organic produce, wild-caught fish, and grass-fed beef.
- Avoid using plastic for food or beverages.

Supplements

- Stop taking the poor-quality men's performance supplement he ordered online.
- Take fish oil (2,000 mg of EPA + DHA combined) to lower LDL cholesterol and increase omega-3 levels (reducing heart disease risk).

- Methylated B-complex vitamin, once per day, to help his body clear dangerous substances (and decrease his risk from toxicity) and replenish Vitamin B deficiencies.
- Acetyl-L-carnitine for brain health.
- Tribulus for stable energy and libido.

Exercise

- Add in more cardio as high-intensity interval training at least three times a week
- Do resistance training at least once a week.
- Do flexibility and core training once a week.

Medication

- No medications indicated.

Stress Management and Sleep

- Engage in daily meditation practice to reduce stress and reactivity. Consider trying an app like Calm, Headspace, or 10% Happier.

Specialists and Complementary Modalities

- Consider acupuncture for helping with stress and cutting back on cravings for sugar.

Of course, this is a lot for Austin to take on all at once. He works with a health coach to plan out which elements to start when, beginning with something that will provide quick results to create a feeling of accomplishment and validation that he's heading in the right direction. They start with exercise, because Austin believes that if he is more active, he'll feel better quickly. They schedule his five workouts per week, each under an hour, into his calendar.

After two weeks on this program, he reports in to his coach. He is on track with 80 percent of his exercise days, and he is ready to work on his diet. He meets with a nutritionist to discuss his schedule, what his tastes are, and how to deal with situations when he's likely to drink too much alcohol or eat too much sugar.

After another two weeks, Austin has his exercise regimen set, and he is feeling good with his meal plan. He downloads a mindfulness app and starts checking it out.

By working with his set program, Austin can benefit by incorporating a wearable that tracks his activity, sleep, stress levels (by measuring his heart rate variability), and food intake (for many apps, all he has to do is take pictures of what he eats). This way, with his permission, a coach and nutritionist can check in and offer him feedback on his choices. He chose as his primary outcomes of interest his general level of energy and his focus at 4:00 p.m. So every day at that time, he gets a reminder to record his level of energy and his level of mental focus on scales of 1 to 10. This allows the coach and nutritionist to use his data to help determine what may be contributing to particularly good or bad days, and provide feedback. They notice bad days are usually related to Austin not sleeping well.

We analyze Austin's data in real time, allowing me to tweak his plan according to how he's feeling, how he's sleeping, his response to exercise, his weight, and his stress levels. The app utilizes machine learning to enable me to provide Austin with more personalized recommendations for diet (which particular foods seem to affect him negatively, for example), supplements (he gets no real benefit from the original Tribulus energy formula based on exercise and stress measurements, but we find another one that does work well for him).

All of this enables us to provide a truly customized dynamic blueprint for Austin to follow so that he can stay on his game and be healthy. Sure enough, after three months, Austin feels physically strong and mentally fit, and he looks great. He has the energy to follow his plan and perform his job as well as interview co-founders for his start-up.

Precision Prevention: The Future of Optimized Health

Austin's case highlights several key elements of a precision prevention plan, which is the future of truly optimized health for men. The particular tests and recommendations we chose for Austin are not important; rather, the point is that we are individualizing testing based on your unique risks for health problems as determined by your own history, genetics, and goals. From this, a picture emerges of where problems could appear down the road. Based on test results, your healthcare provider can provide you with your own precision prevention blueprint that includes medications, supplements, a diet plan, exercise recommendations, stress management tools, sleep optimizers, and recommendations for specialty care.

I emphasize that this is the future goal for optimal health. There are not a lot of providers yet trained in this approach, but the more you ask for it, the more practitioners will get trained in this proactive way. And you don't necessarily need an expensive trainer, coach, or nutritionist. There are inexpensive wearable devices and apps to help you track progress, set goals, monitor what is working for you, and hold yourself accountable.[2]

This personalized plan provides accountability. You can gain accountability through the support of a health coach (which can be a virtual one accessed through your smartphone) and by setting measurable goals, such as weight loss, losing inches from the waist, or improved fitness measurements. Monitoring achievement of goals helps you to stay on track and feel a sense of accomplishment along the way. Involving the support of like-minded guys, as well as a bit of friendly competition, helps to keep you motivated to continue to move forward with healthy behaviors, such as a new exercise program. This combination of community and competition is found in many online social competition groups such as Strava or MapMyRun.

Elements of Precision Prevention

- Personalized health risk assessment
- Analysis of risks in context of goals
- Integrative medicine blue print for health
- Monitoring of progress for accountability
- Health coach support
- Social competition

The individualized approach helps men better understand why there are so many varying, and oftentimes conflicting, recommendations out there for the "best" diet, supplements, or exercise program. Everyone has unique needs, so what works for your friend may not work for you, even if you have similar goals, because of your unique health history and genes. Having advanced testing that identifies your individual characteristics helps you understand why your customized blueprint would be unique.

Advanced testing, wearable technology feeding back data, a clear plan for optimal health that changes according to such data coming in, and the use of health coaches will be the cornerstones of this approach to optimal men's health. This is not necessarily all available widely now, and when it is, it can be expensive, but it will become more broadly available and covered by insurance. Look out for specific interventions utilizing supplements that support brain health (nootropics), stem cells, 3-D printing of biologic tissue, and truly personalized therapies to become part of such personalized approaches to staying healthy.

Eight Levers of Optimal Health

- Medical
- Nutrition and supplements
- Behaviors
- Stress and emotions
- Social
- Physical activity
- Spiritual
- Environment

In the meantime, it is up to you to take your health into your own hands. Remember the eight levers of optimal health—and only one of them centers on medications. There are so many more tools ready for you to use in your quest toward optimal health in service of your optimal life.

Notes

1. This approach aiming to identify personalized risks for health problems can include labs available through a traditional primary care provider, but many primary care providers are not trained in advanced testing. This approach is easier to find from an integrative or functional medicine provider. Unfortunately, many integrative or functional physicians are out-of-network, meaning they don't accept insurance. Therefore throughout the book I have included recommended tests that you can ask your primary care provider to order. I can't guarantee these tests would all be covered by insurance. You have to check with your health plan about specific coverage.

2. Examples of devices that can help you track progress related to exercise, diet, sleep and stress include:

   - Apple Health Kit, available on iPhones and the Apple Watch (able to track activity well)
   - Fitbit wearable trackers (able to track activity especially well)
   - Garmin watches (some models track sleep as well as activity)
   - Oura ring (excellent at tracking stress, activity, and especially sleep quality and quantity)
   - Whoop (a wearable wristband that tracks sleep, activity, and stress, providing a measure of overall strain)

About the Author

Myles Spar, MD, MPH is board certified in Integrative and Internal Medicine and on the academic faculty of the University of California Los Angeles (UCLA) and University of Arizona Schools of Medicine. He has been awarded the highest honor in integrative medicine by his peers and has presented internationally on his dual passions of integrative men's health and bringing holistic, patient-empowered care to the underserved. Dr. Spar consults with professional athletes, executives, and organizations and serves as chief medical officer for Vault Health, Inc., a company dedicated to equipping men with optimal health. His belief in staying healthy in order to win underlies everything he does from being a father of twins and husband to being an Ironman triathlete and informs all of the content he provides through his website, DrSpar.com.

Index

Page numbers followed by *b*, *f*, and *t* refer to boxes, figures, and tables, respectively.

For the benefit of digital users, indexed terms that span two pages (e.g., 52–53) may, on occasion, appear on only one of those pages.

Index

Index

Index

Index